Dear Reader,

Pre-diabetes is something to take seriously, but not fear. Whether you have just received a diagnosis or you have known for some time, you probably realize that lifestyle changes are wise steps toward a **healthier future**. *The Everything® Easy Pre-Diabetes Cookbook* is designed to guide and motivate you along your journey to embrace a more nutritious way of preparing and eating food as well as adopting self-care practices for a lifetime.

Despite what you may have heard, there is no need to eliminate carbs or go "keto" to control blood sugar. As a dietitian in private practice for twenty-five years, I have worked with many clients with pre-diabetes. Almost always, people expect that they need to eliminate all of their most beloved foods and follow a strict diet. I promise, that is not true! Fortunately, after learning how to adapt some of their eating and lifestyle choices, most are pleasantly surprised how **easy and tasty** it is. I don't believe in never-ever foods, and eating should not cause feelings of guilt or shame. Managing pre-diabetes is about common sense and moderation, not deprivation. Perfection is not necessary, as even small changes can result in positive health benefits.

This cookbook contains a wide array of recipes. Some are modern makeovers of old standbys and others will be completely new or different, which means there are lots of fun ways to **explore and create new cooking habits**. I encourage you to expand your food choices and variety while also embracing my pro tips and applying them to your own favorite recipes.

Empowering people to take control of their health warms my heart. When recipes result in great-tasting foods, cooking becomes a pleasure. It is my sincere hope that this book serves as a partner on your journey to better health and well-being. I'm cheering you on!

Think healthy, not skinny,
Lauren Harris-Pincus, MS, RDN

Welcome to the Everything® Series!

These handy, accessible books give you all you need to tackle a difficult project, gain a new hobby, comprehend a fascinating topic, prepare for an exam, or even brush up on something you learned back in school but have since forgotten.

You can choose to read an Everything® book from cover to cover or just pick out the information you want from our four useful boxes: Questions, Facts, Alerts, and Essentials. We give you everything you need to know on the subject, but throw in a lot of fun stuff along the way too.

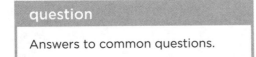

question

Answers to common questions.

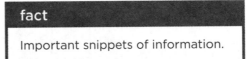

fact

Important snippets of information.

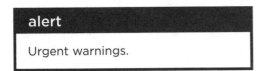

alert

Urgent warnings.

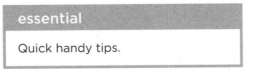

essential

Quick handy tips.

We now have more than 600 Everything® books in print, spanning such wide-ranging categories as cooking, health, parenting, personal finance, wedding planning, word puzzles, and so much more. When you're done reading them all, you can finally say you know Everything®!

PUBLISHER Karen Cooper

MANAGING EDITOR Lisa Laing

COPY CHIEF Casey Ebert

PRODUCTION EDITOR Jo-Anne Duhamel

ACQUISITIONS EDITOR Rachael Thatcher

SENIOR DEVELOPMENT EDITOR Brett Palana-Shanahan

EVERYTHING® SERIES COVER DESIGNER Erin Alexander

THE
EVERYTHING®
EASY
PRE-
DIABETES
COOKBOOK

LAUREN HARRIS-PINCUS, MS, RDN

**200 HEALTHY RECIPES TO HELP
REVERSE AND MANAGE PRE-DIABETES**

ADAMS MEDIA

NEW YORK   LONDON   TORONTO   SYDNEY   NEW DELHI

For my mom, Marilyn, my cooking role model and eager recipe tester.
Your unconditional and unwavering love and support means everything.
Mimi would be kvelling!

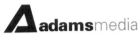

Adams Media
An Imprint of Simon & Schuster, Inc.
100 Technology Center Drive
Stoughton, Massachusetts 02072

Copyright © 2021 by Simon & Schuster, Inc.

All rights reserved, including the right to reproduce this book or portions thereof in any form whatsoever. For information address Adams Media Subsidiary Rights Department, 1230 Avenue of the Americas, New York, NY 10020.

An Everything® Series Book.
Everything® and everything.com® are registered trademarks of Simon & Schuster, Inc.

First Adams Media trade paperback edition October 2021

ADAMS MEDIA and colophon are trademarks of Simon & Schuster.

For information about special discounts for bulk purchases, please contact Simon & Schuster Special Sales at 1-866-506-1949 or business@simonandschuster.com.

The Simon & Schuster Speakers Bureau can bring authors to your live event. For more information or to book an event contact the Simon & Schuster Speakers Bureau at 1-866-248-3049 or visit our website at www.simonspeakers.com.

Interior design by Colleen Cunningham
Photographs by James Stefiuk

Manufactured in the United States of America

4 2023

Library of Congress Cataloging-in-Publication Data has been applied for.

ISBN 978-1-5072-1655-2
ISBN 978-1-5072-1656-9 (ebook)

Many of the designations used by manufacturers and sellers to distinguish their products are claimed as trademarks. Where those designations appear in this book and Simon & Schuster, Inc., was aware of a trademark claim, the designations have been printed with initial capital letters.

MyPlate image © United States Department of Agriculture.

Always follow safety and commonsense cooking protocols while using kitchen utensils, operating ovens and stoves, and handling uncooked food. If children are assisting in the preparation of any recipe, they should always be supervised by an adult.

This book is intended as general information only, and should not be used to diagnose or treat any health condition. In light of the complex, individual, and specific nature of health problems, this book is not intended to replace professional medical advice. The ideas, procedures, and suggestions in this book are intended to supplement, not replace, the advice of a trained medical professional. Consult your physician before adopting any of the suggestions in this book, as well as about any condition that may require diagnosis or medical attention. The author and publisher disclaim any liability arising directly or indirectly from the use of this book.

Contains material adapted from the following titles published by Adams Media, an Imprint of Simon & Schuster, Inc.: *The Everything® Pre-Diabetes Cookbook* by Gretchen Scalpi, RD, CDN, CDE, copyright © 2014, ISBN 978-1-4405-7223-4; *The Everything® Easy DASH Diet Cookbook* by Christy Ellingsworth and Murdoc Khaleghi, MD, copyright © 2021, ISBN 978-1-5072-1521-0; *The Everything® Guide to the Insulin Resistance Diet* by Marie Feldman, RD, CDCES, and Jodi Dalyai, MS, RD, CDCES, copyright © 2021, ISBN 978-1-5072-1420-6.

Contents

Acknowledgments

Writing this book during the Covid-19 pandemic stirred up a wide range of emotions. My heart goes out to everyone affected, whether physically, emotionally, or financially. Self-care took a backseat for so many of us during this time and I hope this book will serve as a motivator to ease back into taking control of our health and well-being.

Many thanks to Beth Shepard, my fabulous agent and friend for believing in me and skipping down the publishing road with me for the second time! To Rachael Thatcher, Lisa Laing, and the entire team at Simon and Schuster for your expertise and for patiently supporting me throughout this enormous project.

To my mom and dad for their lifelong unconditional love and support. To my sister, Julie, for the plant-based cooking inspiration. To my husband, Allan, for nurturing my dream eggs and encouraging me to follow my winding and exciting entrepreneurial path. To my not-so-little loves, Jared and Jordan; the lights of my life, it's an honor to be your mom. Thank you for the always-appreciated and much-needed creative input, tech support, and hugs on demand. Love you "infinite"!

Introduction

If you are reading this cookbook, it's likely you have concerns about the fact that you or a loved one has pre-diabetes. Once diagnosed with pre-diabetes, most people realize that they need to take action in order to gain control of the situation. Fortunately, *The Everything® Easy Pre-Diabetes Cookbook* is here to make life on a diabetes-friendly diet easy and delicious.

Being diagnosed with pre-diabetes means your blood sugar is higher than normal, but it's not high enough to be considered type 2 diabetes. It's important to remember that pre-diabetes doesn't guarantee a progression to type 2 diabetes. One of the most important things you can do to get your health on track is to embrace a healthy, balanced diet with appropriate portions and combinations of foods to help stabilize blood sugar.

This doesn't mean you need to wave goodbye to the dishes you love. Small changes can make a big difference. You'll see that the two hundred recipes in this book are delicious and may feature healthy swaps or tweaks to your favorite foods. Love pizza? You'll be thrilled to see the Buffalo Chicken Flatbread in Chapter 3. If you're partial to Chinese food, check out the Hoisin Chicken Lettuce Wraps in Chapter 4. And for the pasta lovers out there, try out the Fresh Tomato and Clam Sauce with Whole-Grain Linguine in Chapter 8.

The recipes you'll find in the pages to come are nutritious and tasty in addition to being both quick and easy to make. No master chef skills are needed here. The good news is that every recipe in this book can be made in 30 minutes or less, eliminating the need to sacrifice time in the name of health. Let this guide take some of that stress off your plate.

In this cookbook you'll find practical information to empower you to learn about a healthier way of preparing and eating food. It can be hard, but don't give up! Your body will thank you! Taking control means creating an action plan that fits into your lifestyle. You have been given an opportunity to prevent or delay the onset of type 2 diabetes. Embrace it!

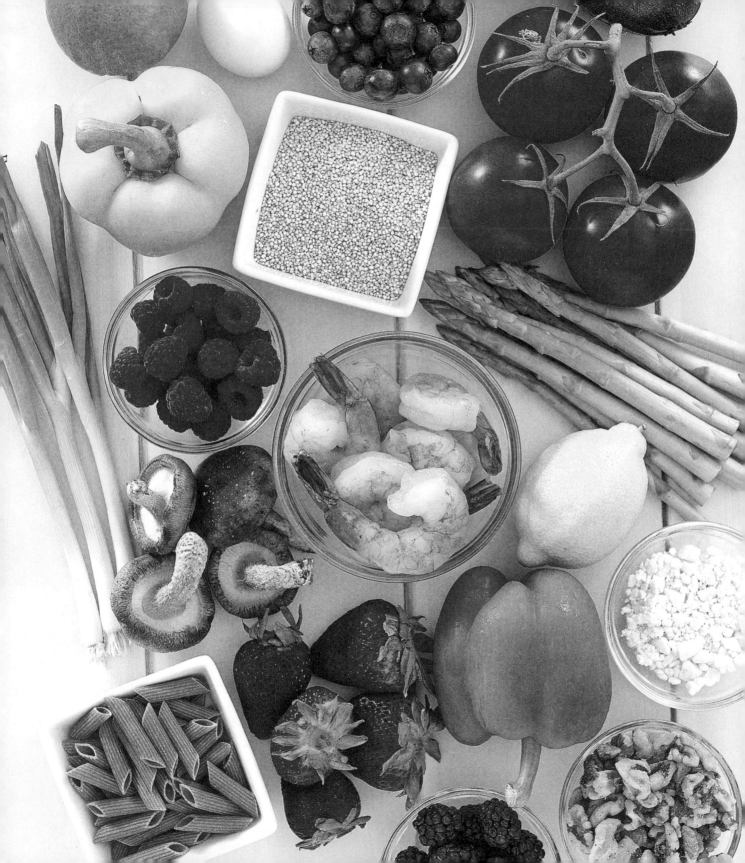

CHAPTER 1

Managing and Reversing Pre-Diabetes

Your doctor has just told you that you have, or your loved one has, pre-diabetes. Your initial reaction might have been shock, anger, or a feeling of helplessness. Perhaps you knew something was not quite right all along, but you tried to put the whole thing out of your mind. Whatever the case, you are now faced with a medical diagnosis that has the potential to be serious if ignored. Many people in this situation do not know what pre-diabetes means or what to do about it. You can start by learning more about pre-diabetes and taking steps to stop pre-diabetes in its tracks.

What Is Pre-Diabetes?

The most recent data from the National Diabetes Statistics Report, 2020, put out by the Centers for Disease Control and Prevention (CDC), estimates that as of 2018, there were 88 million Americans with pre-diabetes. Yes, you read that correctly: 88 million people—that's 1 in 3 Americans! The numbers are growing annually, in large part because pre-diabetes is linked to America's other serious health problems—an increasing rate of overweight and obesity. Having an elevated body fat mass and elevated blood sugar tend to go hand in hand, as evidenced by 89 percent of those diagnosed with pre-diabetes. Blood sugar that fluctuates too high or too low throughout the day has a direct influence on your hunger level and snacking habits. If your blood sugar is too low, you may eat too much food. If you consume calories in excess of what you need, over time you gain weight. Weight gain can set the stage for developing pre-diabetes, which, if left unchecked, can lead to diabetes.

If you have obesity, your risk for developing pre-diabetes is far greater. Recent data from the CDC indicates that 42.4 percent of adults in the United States have obesity. One very important thing to understand is that obesity is up to 70 percent inherited. There are hundreds of genes that contribute to determining body weight and body fat. Obesity is not a lack of willpower, and simply eating less and moving more will not guarantee a fix. What's key is working with healthcare professionals to determine the right course of action for your body. Often, the number on the scale is not nearly as important as the quality of your diet and lifestyle behaviors. Find a team of practitioners who meet you where you are as a whole person versus focusing only on your weight.

> **fact**
>
> The term "pre-diabetes" was introduced by the American Diabetes Association in 2002 as a way to more clearly convey a state that is between normal blood sugar and type 2 diabetes. The old phrase "borderline diabetes" provides little meaning to the person hearing it, and it certainly does not convey the urgent need to do something about it.

When you have pre-diabetes, your blood sugar level is higher than normal but not yet high enough to be diagnosed as type 2 diabetes. Pre-diabetes means that you are on your way to developing diabetes if there are no interventions on your part. It is important to understand that progression from pre-diabetes to type 2 diabetes is not inevitable. There is a great deal that you can do to reverse pre-diabetes and bring your blood sugar level back to a normal range.

Pre-diabetes is a wake-up call that gives you an opportunity to improve your health and make healthy lifestyle changes. If you take action now, you can prevent, or at the very least, delay progression to serious, diabetes-related complications. Small changes can make a big difference.

Your Action Plan for Pre-Diabetes

Taking steps to stop the progression of pre-diabetes is necessary to restore good health. With pre-diabetes, there is still a chance for you to prevent the onset of type 2 diabetes. Even if you develop diabetes eventually at a later time, slowing down the progression will result in fewer complications.

There are three essential components to your action plan:

- If needed, losing weight and keeping it off (even a small reduction can yield benefits)
- Eating healthier by improving eating habits
- Maintaining consistent physical activity

It is important to develop an action plan to help you make lifestyle changes gradually. Have no more than two or three specific, tangible goals to work on at one time. This strategy prevents you from becoming overwhelmed and allows you to master a goal before moving on to something else. Also, try a small reward system for goals achieved—something not related to food—to keep you motivated and to celebrate your success!

Losing Weight

An elevated body weight may be only one of several contributors to pre-diabetes; however, it is one factor that may be helped by lifestyle modifications. Body mass index (BMI) is one piece of information healthcare practitioners can use to determine how your weight is categorized.

- A BMI of 18.5–24.9 = normal weight
- A BMI of 25–29.9 = overweight
- A BMI of 30 or greater = Class I obesity

Your doctor can tell you what your BMI is, or you can use the BMI calculator at www.nhlbi.nih.gov/health/educational/lose_wt/BMI/bmicalc.htm to determine this yourself. Your weight is influenced by many genetic and environmental factors and should only be used as a data point, not to judge or blame yourself for your choices.

The good news is there are many rewards that come with modest weight loss. There is no need to set unrealistic goals. According to the 2019 consensus report on *Nutrition*

Therapy for Adults with Diabetes or Prediabetes, the goal is a 7–10 percent weight loss for preventing progression to type 2 diabetes. That means weight loss of as little as 10–20 pounds can prevent or delay development of diabetes. Modest weight loss also helps reduce insulin resistance, cholesterol levels, and blood pressure.

People who have advanced to type 2 diabetes gradually lose the ability to make adequate amounts of insulin. When this happens, weight loss and exercise alone are not enough to control blood glucose. Medications are often a necessary part of treatment, and research is showing that earlier intervention with medication and lifestyle changes can better prevent progression to type 2 diabetes.

Eating Healthier

Contrary to popular belief, sugar isn't toxic or poisonous, and you don't get diabetes from eating too much sugar. However, too much sugar can crowd out nutritious food, meaning that for the calorie level your body needs, there's not enough room for the important nutrients required to function optimally. Too much sugar also provides empty calories, which in the end can cause weight gain. Weight gain in turn can increase insulin resistance, which can result in prediabetes developing into diabetes.

Change your mindset from one of restriction to one of addition. Focus on what you can add to your diet versus what you think you should eliminate. The quality of your diet and how you view your food are both important factors in success. Consuming more fruits, vegetables, beans, and whole grains will increase fiber intake and fill you up so there is less room for higher-calorie, nutrient-poor foods. **There is no such thing as a never-ever food**. The key is twofold: First, identify choices that will enhance your health; and second, identify those choices that have the potential to curb your progress—and then work on ways to reduce your exposure to them.

Make your food environment friendly and keep it stocked with plant-based food choices. Try to also minimize foods that tempt you to overconsume and thereby take in unnecessary calories. Start by reviewing the foods you routinely buy at the grocery store. Are these foods helping you reach your goals or are they self-sabotaging? What kinds of foods are in your kitchen?

Many people have a hard time cleaning up their food environment because of other people living in the household. Keeping less healthy foods in the house for others is not likely to help you stay on track. Remember that healthy eating is important for everyone, and having trigger foods around the house makes it difficult to resist eating those foods. Discuss your concerns with your family and come to a compromise on how often these foods should be brought into the household. It's not fair to expect yourself to rely on willpower to avoid eating irresistible foods.

Make your food environment supportive by keeping nutritious food and snack alternatives available at all times. At the grocery store, be sure to purchase healthy snack items for everyone in the family. When they are readily available, it becomes easier to avoid the impulsiveness of problematic food decisions.

Snacks should be balanced with protein- and fiber-rich foods to help balance blood sugar. They are a great time to include extra fruit and vegetables into your day. Keep snacks in the range of 100–200 calories, and make sure to combine some protein, fiber-rich carbs, and healthy fats. Here are a few examples:

- Carrot sticks with 2 tablespoons hummus
- Low-fat mozzarella cheese stick and a small piece of fruit
- 1 tablespoon peanut butter with a small apple
- 6 ounces plain or low-sugar Greek yogurt with ½ cup berries and a few nuts

Getting Started with Exercise

Exercise is an important part of your action plan for halting pre-diabetes. The role of physical activity cannot be underestimated! Regular movement will improve your blood glucose levels, which is achieved when the glucose in blood is used for energy during and after exercise. Muscle cells become more sensitive to insulin, and insulin resistance improves. Gradually blood glucose levels go down.

First, talk to your doctor to make sure that exercise is appropriate for you. In most cases, your doctor will support your desire to engage in physical activity. If you have other health issues in addition to pre-diabetes, you and your doctor will want to discuss the best types of activity for you. Once you have the okay to start, it's useful to consider what type of exercise will be beneficial for you:

- Consider your physical ability and choose activities that you can do.
- Include activities you enjoy or those you already do on a regular basis. Walking, gardening, and house cleaning are all ways to get exercise.
- Think about how much time you have for exercise. A fitness plan that takes too much time will quickly be abandoned if it's too ambitious.
- Consider the resources available. If you do not have access to a gym, exercise equipment, or a pool, then walking may be your best bet. With online streaming services, a fitness class is only a click away and not dependent on the weather. Love

to dance? Put on some tunes and go for it. Exercise does not need to be organized to be effective, and joyful movement is the best kind.

When planning your exercise routine, be honest about whether you will maintain the plan. Can you perform the activity outdoors year-round or will you need to find an alternative indoor activity for part of the year? Is it appropriate for your physical capabilities and fitness level? Before you start, work through any barriers that could get in the way of your success. Short periods of time (ten to thirty minutes) will probably work much better than trying to carve out an hour for daily activity. Here are ways to slip in activity every day without making huge demands on your schedule:

- Park farther away from your destination, and then walk the rest of the way.
- During the workday, get up from your desk to walk or stretch every hour.

- If you have access to stairs, walk up and down a flight or two several times per day.
- Consider using a standing desk or a treadmill desk to fit more movement into your workday.
- Go for a ten-minute walk after lunch or dinner.
- Stand or walk in place while you are on the telephone or watching TV.

For most people, walking is a good place to begin because it is easy and requires no special equipment other than a pair of good walking shoes. Walking three times a week for ten to fifteen minutes at a time can help ease you into a regular routine. As you become stronger and gain more endurance, gradually increase your walking time by five minutes every week, until you are able to walk for a full thirty minutes at a time. Once you can walk for thirty minutes, increase your frequency to four or five times weekly. Brisk walking is an aerobic exercise and an effective strategy for controlling blood sugar. Plus, you can bring along a friend, family member, or even your dog to make your fitness journey more enjoyable. Find an accountability buddy to keep you honest and motivated.

Consistent exercise benefits everyone, especially if you have pre-diabetes. While diabetes prevention is at the top of the list, you may also enjoy lower blood pressure, lower lipid levels, reduced stress, and better sleep.

Once you have had success with maintaining exercise, find new ways to get active and keep it interesting. Varying the routine helps to keep you from getting bored, and it challenges your body in different ways. Your exercise program should be one that you can maintain for life. Think of your exercise program as a work in progress by finding new ways to improve it and keep it fun. Slow, steady progress will help you achieve your goals!

Balance and Moderation Are Key

You may think that having pre-diabetes means you will have to give up everything you like to eat. Nothing could be further from the truth! With the help and advice of a registered dietitian, you can develop healthy eating habits that fit into your lifestyle.

Try to think of changes in your eating habits as goals rather than inflexible rules. Start by making a list of the things you would like to change or improve. Decide exactly what you need to do in order to bring about change, and then select one or two changes to work on at a time. Here are a few ideas to help you start this process:

- Eat meals at regular intervals (every four to five hours). Resolve not to skip meals or go for long periods of time without eating, except possibly between dinner and bedtime.
- Include nutritious snacks in your daily eating plan. Hint: Snacks are a great way to include more fruits and vegetables into your daily diet!
- Start reducing your portion sizes. Cut back by 25–30 percent to get used to eating less. Using the plate method as a guide can be very helpful to help control helpings without counting calories. At meals, try to eat ½ of your food volume from fruits and vegetables, ¼ from lean proteins, and ¼ from whole grains, beans, and starchy vegetables.
- Drink plenty of water every day. Most adults need at least 48–64 ounces daily.

Everyone should eat a healthy diet regardless of whether or not they have pre-diabetes. You may be surprised to learn that your plan will have the same foods that everyone else should eat and that buying diet foods is usually unnecessary. You may wish to use noncaloric sweeteners or certain sugar-free foods to add variety; this is not essential, but you may find it helpful if you like sweet foods and wish to limit your intake of added sugars. You will not have to prepare one meal for yourself and something different for the rest of your family. The recipes in this cookbook use ingredients suitable for everyone. To put it simply, a meal plan for managing pre-diabetes is a healthy plan that most people can follow.

Carbohydrates and Pre-Diabetes

Carbohydrates serve as the body's primary energy source. Simple carbohydrates include sugars, sweets, juices, and fruits. Complex carbohydrates include all types of grain products and starchy vegetables such as potatoes, peas, and corn. Recommendations for a healthy diet suggest that most carbohydrates come from the complex carbohydrates rather than simple sugars. Complex carbohydrates found in whole-grain foods provide better nutritional value and are a source of vitamins, minerals, and fiber. Fruit contains natural simple sugars, and they are also sources of essential nutrients. **People with prediabetes do not need to avoid fruit!** In fact, a recent study in *The Journal of Clinical Endocrinology and Metabolism* found an association between consuming whole fruit and improved insulin sensitivity, suggesting people who consumed more fruit had to produce less insulin to lower blood sugar levels. To get the most fiber from fruit, choose fresh, frozen, or unsweetened canned or dried fruit instead of fruit juice.

Research shows that 95 percent of Americans fall short of the recommended fiber intake of 14 grams per 1,000 calories, which roughly equals 25 grams for women and 38 grams for men per day. Fiber can be a key ally in fighting pre-diabetes. We get fiber from plant foods such as fruits, vegetables, whole grains, legumes, nuts, beans, and seeds. Make these the basis of your overall diet to increase the amount of fiber you consume.

Having pre-diabetes does not mean you must cut out all carbohydrates from your diet. Choose carbohydrates that have good nutritional value and maintain an appropriate portion size. The amount of carbohydrates each person needs is very individualized and is primarily determined by your body size and activity level. Appetite and hunger also play an important role, and meal timing and combining can affect how your body responds to the carbs you consume. There is no magic number, so refrain from comparing yourself to others when trying to figure out what is best for you. To best determine how many carbs you should be eating, schedule an appointment with a registered dietitian. They will work with you to create an eating plan specific to your personal, medical, financial, cultural, and culinary needs. And most insurance companies cover these services, so it may be free to you!

---

question

What are whole grains?

The Food and Drug Administration (FDA) has defined whole grains as "the intact, ground, cracked, or flaked fruit of the grains whose principal components—the starchy endosperm, germ, and bran—are present in the same relative proportions as they exist in the intact grain." In other words, no part of the grain has been removed during processing, so you are getting all parts of the grain.

Proteins: Building Blocks to Good Health

Proteins are the building blocks of the body and are used for growth, building, and repair. Despite what you may have heard, more is not necessarily better. Your plan can include lean sources of meat, fish, poultry, eggs, and milk products. Plant-based proteins are found in nuts, seeds, and legumes (beans and lentils). While most Americans consume enough total protein, it's important to distribute it evenly throughout the day to maintain muscle mass as we age, which supports our metabolism. We can only absorb and utilize 25–35 grams of protein per meal for muscle growth and repair. Breakfast is a time where protein is often underconsumed, and this cannot be made up later in the day by doubling up on protein at afternoon or evening meals. Aim for at least 20 grams of protein at breakfast.

Fats: Monos, Polys, Saturated, and Trans

All fats, regardless of type, have a significant number of calories—about 100–120 calories per tablespoon for most types. Therefore, moderation of any fat is recommended. Every gram of fat contains 9 calories.

Monounsaturated fat should make up most of the fat you consume. This type of fat is found in plant foods such as walnuts, avocado, canola oil, peanut oil, and olive oil. Monounsaturated fat does not raise blood cholesterol and may actually help reduce blood cholesterol levels if it replaces saturated fat in the diet.

Polyunsaturated fat should be consumed in moderation and less often than monounsaturated fat. This fat comes mostly from vegetable sources such as corn oil, sunflower oil, and some types of margarine. These are most often found in processed foods like chips and crackers.

---

essential

Check food labels and ingredients to avoid trans fat as much as possible. This form of fat can raise LDL (bad) cholesterol and increase your risk for heart disease. Trans fat can be found in vegetable shortenings, solid margarines, certain crackers and cookies, and other foods made with partially hydrogenated oils. These are found far less in foods today after the FDA instituted rules about trans fat content, but most of the time they are found in highly processed foods.

Saturated fat should be used the least. This type of fat is found in animal-source foods such as meat, butter, and cheese. Baked goods may be high in saturated fat if lard, palm oil, or coconut oil is used. Excessive intake of saturated fat can increase blood cholesterol levels.

Cholesterol

Cholesterol is a waxy substance found in all body cells. The liver makes much of the cholesterol your body needs, but cholesterol is also obtained from the foods you eat.

Cholesterol is found in animal foods such as meat, eggs, butter, and whole dairy products.

Too much cholesterol in the blood can increase your risk for heart disease. However, there isn't a direct correlation between the amount of cholesterol you consume from food and levels of blood cholesterol. It's the saturated fat content of the food that is more directly correlated to increasing cholesterol levels. This is often confusing when it comes to foods like eggs and shellfish that are naturally higher in cholesterol. Eating eggs in moderation should be fine for most people, as is shellfish like shrimp, crab, and lobster. It is recommended to limit consumption of fatty meats, butter, full-fat dairy foods and tropical oils like palm and coconut oil.

Sodium

Sodium is a mineral that does not affect blood sugar, but it can alter your blood pressure. Keeping blood pressure under control is an important aspect of managing pre-diabetes and preventing heart disease. Here are some tips for reducing sodium:

- Leave out or reduce the amount of salt in standard recipes by 25–50 percent.
- To reduce the sodium content of dishes, salt it at the end—that way you will taste it directly versus dispersed through the food.
- Use commercial herb blends or make your own to season food instead of using salt.
- Limit processed foods when possible such as boxed mixes, TV dinners, and processed meats. If necessary, there are some lower-sodium versions available.
- Make more meals and side dishes from scratch.
- Watch your use of the saltshaker in cooking or at the table.

Food Combining and Timing Matters

Most foods are not eaten alone. The rise in blood sugar from consuming carbohydrates will be affected by what accompanies them. A balanced meal of protein, high-fiber carbohydrates, and healthy fats will take longer to digest and blunt a rise in blood sugar versus choosing a bagel with jelly or a soft hot pretzel, which are almost entirely carbohydrate-based. Each meal and snack should contain protein, carbohydrates, and some fat for better blood sugar control.

The order in which you eat your foods can matter as well. If you have a plate of grilled chicken, rice, and sautéed broccoli, research shows that eating the rice toward the end will raise blood sugar less than eating it earlier in the meal. Basically, having the protein and fiber in your stomach first will delay the digestion of the rice more than if you eat it earlier. Simple adjustments in how you eat can make a difference—even without weight loss.

About Fiber and Whole Grains

There are two types of fiber found in foods—soluble and insoluble—and each behaves differently in the body. It's important to include foods containing both types of fiber in your daily eating plan. Foods like beans, barley, and oats are especially good sources of a type of soluble fiber that can form a gel and help to bind some glucose and cholesterol. Vegetables, whole-grain foods, and fruit are all sources of insoluble fiber. Another type of fiber is called resistant starch, which is resistant to digestion and serves as food for the good bacteria that live in your colon. It is formed when pasta, rice, and potatoes are cooked and then cooled, which means leftovers of these foods will have less effect on blood sugar than freshly cooked versions.

fact

The terms multigrain, seven-grain, and stone-ground do not necessarily mean a product is whole-grain. If a whole-grain ingredient is not listed as the first ingredient, the item may contain only a small portion of whole grains. One way to find a whole-grain product is to look for the Whole Grains Council stamp of approval, which labels foods containing whole grains. The logo that reads "100% Whole Grain" indicates that the food has only whole grains and at least 16g per serving. Note that grams of whole grain and grams of fiber are not the same. A 16g serving of a whole grain may contain anywhere from 0.6–2.9 grams of fiber depending on the food, with brown rice on the low end and bulgur or barley on the high end.

Although all types of grains are sources of complex carbohydrates, those that have not been refined are better for you. Whole grains have not had the bran layer and germ removed during the milling process; therefore, the fiber as well as vitamins and minerals are preserved. Fiber helps to slow down the absorption of glucose into the bloodstream, which helps to keep blood glucose controlled. Refined grains such as white-flour products have the bran and germ removed, making them much lower in fiber. Whenever you can, choose whole grains over refined grains, they are not lower in calories but are better options for helping to control blood sugar.

Great Ways to Get More Whole Grains

The best way to get more whole grains in your meals is to substitute whole-grain foods for refined products. Here are some tips:

- Instead of all-purpose flour, experiment by replacing some of the flour with a whole-grain version. White whole-wheat flour is a variety that is more pleasing to the palate than whole-wheat flour and can be used in any recipe calling for wheat flour. White whole wheat comes from the white species of wheat that is lighter in color and milder in flavor than red wheat, which is used for traditional whole-wheat flour. However, the nutritional content and fiber are quite similar.
- Use a whole grain as a side dish or combine it with vegetables or beans.
- Try a "new" grain that you have not used before. Quinoa, bulgur, sorghum, farro, black rice, or kasha may be unfamiliar, but they are as easy to prepare as white rice.

- Add whole grains to soups, salads, or casseroles instead of white rice or pasta. If you don't like 100 percent whole-grain pasta, mix it with regular pasta or a fiber-enriched variety to pump up the nutrients and fiber.
- Gradually replace the refined grains in your pantry with whole-grain foods.

Learn How to Read Food Labels

The Nutrition Facts found on food labels contain information, but unless you understand how to read the labels, this information may not mean very much to you. Here are some of the items listed on the Nutrition Facts label:

- **Serving size:** Labels must identify the size of a serving. The nutritional information listed on a label is based on one serving of the food. Take note that a package that seems like a single serving may contain more than one portion. Read the label to make sure.
- **Amount per serving:** Each package identifies the quantities of nutrients and food constituents in one serving. This includes the caloric value of the food, as well as the amount of fat, cholesterol, sodium, carbohydrates, fiber, sugars, added sugars, and protein per serving.
- **Percent daily value:** This indicates how much of a specific nutrient a serving of food contains based on an average 2,000-calorie diet.

- **Ingredients list:** This is a list of the ingredients in a food in descending order of predominance and weight.

Grams of Carbohydrate or Grams of Sugar?

There are several parts to the carbohydrate section of the nutrition label. Total Carbohydrate represents the full amount of carbohydrate grams found in a food. Beneath the Total Carbohydrate are other listings: Fiber, Sugars, Added Sugars, and sometimes Sugar Alcohols. It is important to know that all of these are part of Total Carbohydrate though they have differing effects on blood sugar since all carbohydrates are not created equal.

FIBER

Look for foods where the fiber content is a larger percentage of total carbohydrate. The Dietary Guidelines for Americans recommends a minimum of 14 grams per 1,000 calories, which works out to roughly 25 grams per day for women and 38 grams for men. Foods with 5 grams of fiber per serving provide an excellent source and equal at least 20 percent of the daily needs for women and 13 percent for men.

SUGARS

Since the updated Nutrition Facts panel was introduced, sugars are separated into those naturally occurring and added to the product. Items such as milk, plain yogurt, fruit, and vegetables have *naturally occurring sugar*, which will be counted under the sugar total, but not added sugars. For example,

1 cup of milk has 12 grams of sugar from the naturally occurring lactose already present. Those 12 grams will be listed under sugars, but added sugars would be 0.

ADDED SUGARS

Sugars are sometimes added during the processing of foods such as sweetened beverages, cookies, ice cream, cereal, crackers, yogurt, salad dressing, sauces, marinades, and more. These are listed in the ingredients as dextrose, fructose, lactose, table sugar, beet sugar, honey, corn syrup, turbinado, agave, coconut sugar, and more. The American Heart Association recommends limiting added sugars to 24 grams per day for women (6 teaspoons) and 36 grams per day for men (9 teaspoons).

SUGAR ALCOHOLS

Some foods will also have a line for sugar alcohols on the label under Total Carbohydrates. These are sweeteners that contain anywhere from zero to half the calories of regular sugar. Despite their name, they are neither a sugar nor an alcohol. They exist naturally in certain fruits and vegetables, but some are artificial and are included in processed foods to decrease the added sugars. You will likely find sugar alcohols in many foods labeled "sugar free" or "no sugar added." These may include sorbitol, xylitol, mannitol, erythritol, maltitol, isomalt, lactitol, and hydrogenated starch hydrolysates.

Let's Talk about Net Carbs

Some foods, especially processed foods designed to be lower in sugar may list "Net Carbs" on the packaging. This term does not have a legal definition, is not used by the Food and Drug Administration, and is not recognized by the American Diabetes Association. "Net carbs" are anecdotally determined by subtracting any fiber or sugar alcohols on the label from the total carbohydrates to calculate the available or digestible carbs in the product. This is assuming that fiber and sugar alcohols are not absorbed or metabolized, but some are partially digested and therefore still provide calories as well as impact blood sugar.

The equation used to calculate net carbs is not entirely accurate because the contribution of fiber and sugar alcohols to total carbohydrates depends on the types present. The type of fiber or sugar alcohols used is not specified on the nutrition facts label; therefore the effect on blood glucose and potential insulin therapy adjustments cannot be determined properly. The bottom line: Food companies are using this term to market products. That's not necessarily a bad thing, but you must use caution if using net carbs to make decisions about which or how much of a food to consume.

Grocery Lists and Your Kitchen Makeover

Having the right foods on hand is the best way to keep you eating healthier. If you leave things up to chance, you are more likely to impulsively make less desirable choices. Set aside time each week to plan meals and prep what you can in advance. Keep a weekly shopping list visible and handy; when you think of food items you need, write them on your list. Consider what meals and snacks you will need for the coming week.

Fifteen Foods to Always Have On Hand

1. Vegetables: Fresh, frozen, or canned (reduced-sodium)
2. Fruits: Fresh, frozen (unsweetened), or canned (juice- or water-packed)
3. Whole-grain bread, pasta, or crackers
4. Oatmeal and high-fiber (low-sugar) cereals with 4g or more fiber per serving and less than 6g of added sugar
5. Canned beans, dried beans, or lentils
6. Boneless, skinless chicken or turkey breast
7. Eggs, egg substitutes, or egg whites
8. Tuna, salmon, and sardines canned in water
9. Low-fat cheese or cheese sticks
10. Dried herbs and spices
11. Dry-roasted or raw nuts (unsalted)
12. Low-sodium chicken, vegetable, or beef broth
13. Leafy lettuce varieties or bagged mixes using leafy varieties
14. Low-sodium canned tomatoes
15. Nonfat Greek yogurt: plain, vanilla, or low-sugar fruit-flavored

Let your shopping list be your guide at the grocery store and stick to your list as much as possible. Save money by buying seasonal items in bulk and freezing them for later. Minimize food waste by planning a few meals from the same ingredients so everything is used.

Make Over Your Food Supply

Making over your food supply is easy to do. You can gradually phase out foods of lesser nutritional quality and introduce newer ones that have more health benefits. As you run out of certain items, replace them with something new.

SWITCH TO HEALTHIER OPTIONS

Instead of:	Replace with:
Garlic or onion salt	Fresh garlic or onion
Fruit juices	Fresh fruit
All-purpose flour	Whole-grain flour
Vegetable oil	Olive oil or avocado oil
Sour cream	Plain, low-fat Greek yogurt
Buttery snack crackers	Whole-grain crackers
Potato chips	Popcorn (make your own) or roasted bean snacks

Recipe Adjustments for Your New Cooking Style

Your favorite recipes can be adjusted to lower fat, salt, or sugar content, yet still maintain good taste. Some of the recipes found in this cookbook may contain ingredients such as butter or salt in small amounts. These ingredients are usually part of a recipe because they improve the flavor or aid in the baking or cooking process. Many recipes can withstand up to a 50 percent reduction in fat. To replace fat, use plain Greek yogurt, applesauce, mashed ripe banana, or puréed prunes for half of the fat called for in a recipe. If you must eliminate all butter from your diet, most recipes can use olive, canola, or avocado oil as a substitute. When baking bread, cookies, or cakes, salt is usually essential in the leavening process and should not be eliminated.

Using Sugar Substitutes

Sugar substitutes are never mandatory when you have pre-diabetes; however, they can offer options for those who wish to use them. It is challenging to remain within the guidelines for added sugar intake set by the American Heart Association without using some alternative sweeteners, since most added sugars consumed are already in the processed food we eat. Using a "natural" sugar substitute such as stevia, monk fruit, erythritol, or allulose in a recipe can significantly slash sugar content and calories. When using sugar substitutes in baking, keep in mind that sweetness is being added to the food, but other traits unique to a baked product (volume, texture, color) may be altered. Check with the manufacturer on the best ways to use a sugar substitute for baking. This book will typically call for stevia, monk fruit, or erythritol that measure 1:1, meaning you exchange the product equally with the amount of sugar written in the recipe. Some sugar substitutes measure two times as sweet as sugar, so make sure to check the product labeling before using it.

The recipes for baked desserts found in this cookbook have different methods for addressing sugar. Some use small amounts of honey or maple syrup when appropriate. Many recipes use non-nutritive "natural" sweeteners such as stevia, monk fruit, or erythritol. They have a range of densities and flavors and behave differently depending on the recipe. Stevia tends to be lighter and more powder-like, while monk fruit and erythritol are more granular like sugar. The baked goods you will find here work without blending these sweeteners with sugar. Each recipe was written with a specific sweetener suggestion based on the composition of the dish. Certain desserts like cakes are more delicate and likely won't work with 100 percent stevia, monk fruit, or erythritol. As you work with these or with your own recipes, you will learn how to adjust ingredients to get good results. There are also blended products on the market that mix sugar with these alternative sweeteners to offer significantly less sugar for those recipes that work better with real sugar.

If you don't want to use a non-nutritive sweetener, try reducing a standard recipe's sugar content by 25 percent and gradually decrease the amount of sugar each time you make it. Be sure to note whether the properties of the food change in any significant or undesirable ways, then adjust as needed. Use puréed, unsweetened fruit to replace some of the sugar in a recipe.

question

Can sugar be eliminated from my favorite baked dessert?

Maybe. Completely eliminating sugar from baked desserts can be tricky. Although sugar is an empty-calorie food, it does serve as an important ingredient in baked foods. When sugar is reduced or replaced with a non-nutritive sweetener, the result can be very different and not what you were hoping for. The baked item may lack a golden-brown color or have a flavor unlike the original recipe. The newer non-nutritive sweeteners on the market behave more like sugar and in the right amounts may completely replace sugar if desired.

Taste buds are personal. The same way some folks like their coffee black and others prefer four packets of sweetener, recipes need to be adjusted to the individual. Some of you may think the products here are too sweet, others not sweet enough. That's okay. You get to decide how you like it; just play around with the understanding that you cannot take sweetness away, so begin with less and add more as needed.

Cooking Styles

There are many ways to prepare foods that minimize the use of sugar, salt, and fat yet taste good! A little creativity with spices or herbs makes food more flavorful without the addition of extra fat, sodium, or calories. Stir-frying, broiling, pressure cooking, air frying, and slow cooking are examples of techniques that are timesaving and result in healthier food.

Stir-frying uses small amounts of oil to cook foods quickly at a high heat. Foods that work well using this method include vegetables, poultry, meats, fish, and cooked grains. Choose oil that allows for a high cooking temperature such as canola, avocado, or peanut oil. Remember to use as little oil as possible; usually 1–2 teaspoons will do.

Broiling and grilling involve cooking food on a rack to allow fats to drip to a pan or flame below. Most meats, poultry, and fish can be grilled or broiled. Broiling instead of cooking in oil reduces fat and calories.

Meals made in a slow cooker do not require the addition of fat, and slow cooking helps tenderize tougher cuts of meat. Soups, sauces, and stews are just a few examples of items you can cook in a slow cooker.

Pressure cookers and Instant Pots® usually cook food in a fraction of the time and can be lifesavers when cooking things like a whole chicken, dry beans, spaghetti squash, or whole grains that would normally take an hour or more in the oven.

CHAPTER 2

Breakfast and Brunch

Peanut Chip Breakfast Cookie Dough

SERVES 1

Per Serving:

Calories	250
Fat	9g
Saturated Fat	3g
Cholesterol	5mg
Sodium	190mg
Carbohydrates	21g
Fiber	7g
Sugar	6g
Added Sugars	0g
Protein	21g

WHAT ARE CACAO NIBS?

Cacao nibs are cacao beans that have been cracked, fermented, and broken into smaller pieces. As nature's chocolate chips, they are crunchy and packed with antioxidants and fiber. They are usually made without added sugar and have a slight bitterness. If you like dark chocolate that's at least 70 percent cocoa, you will probably like cacao nibs. If not, stick with sugar-free chocolate chips.

Kids and adults alike enjoy a spoonful of cookie dough every now and then. Unfortunately, that comes with a risk of salmonella from raw eggs plus a ton of calories from fat and sugar. This edible "cookie dough" provides the sweet and salty fun flavor combo you crave in a nutrient-rich meal.

½ cup plain nonfat Greek yogurt

3 tablespoons powdered peanut butter

1 packet stevia

⅛ teaspoon vanilla extract

2 tablespoons old-fashioned oats

2½ teaspoons cacao nibs or sugar-free chocolate chips, divided

1 teaspoon chopped peanuts

1. In a medium bowl, combine yogurt, powdered peanut butter, stevia, vanilla, oats, and 2 teaspoons cacao nibs and gently mix.
2. Top with chopped peanuts and remaining ½ teaspoon cacao nibs. Serve.

Berry Vanilla Protein-Packed Cereal Bowl

If you love cereal but find yourself starving an hour later, more protein in your breakfast might be the solution. The secret formula involves stirring protein powder into your milk of choice; the result is sweet milk like the kind that was left in the bowl of sugary cereal when you were a kid. Replace the strawberries with blueberries, raspberries, or a mixture of all three.

2/3 cup high-fiber cereal, such as Fiber One

2 teaspoons chia seeds

1 cup strawberries, chopped

1 cup unsweetened almond milk or milk of choice

3 tablespoons vanilla grass-fed whey protein powder

1/4 teaspoon ground cinnamon

1. In a medium bowl, place cereal, chia seeds, and strawberries.
2. In a 2-cup measuring cup or glass, whisk together milk and protein powder until completely dissolved. Pour over cereal and fruit and stir to combine. Sprinkle with cinnamon and serve.

SERVES 1	
Per Serving:	
Calories	280
Fat	7g
Saturated Fat	0g
Cholesterol	10mg
Sodium	380mg
Carbohydrates	51g
Fiber	25g
Sugar	7g
Added Sugars	0g
Protein	22g

PROTEIN POWDER OPTIONS

There are extensive options for protein powder, and it comes down to personal choice when deciding which to use. Whey has a pleasing flavor and is rich in the amino acid leucine, which is good for post-workout muscle recovery. Plant-based powders such as pea or brown rice protein will thicken and absorb more liquid so the texture will be different. Look for options with few ingredients and sweetened with stevia, monk fruit, or erythritol.

Protein-Packed Oatmeal

SERVES 1

Per Serving:

Calories	190
Fat	8g
Saturated Fat	2g
Cholesterol	185mg
Sodium	280mg
Carbohydrates	19g
Fiber	3g
Sugar	1g
Added Sugars	0g
Protein	10g

TOPPING OPTIONS

Some delicious topping options for this oatmeal if you are looking for something sweet are fruit, chocolate chips, nut butter, or my Cranberry Compote in this chapter. If you are looking for something savory, try sautéed or roasted vegetables, avocado pieces, or a fried egg.

A warm bowl of oatmeal is a delicious and satisfying way to begin the day, but it lacks the protein needed to help keep you full for hours and balance blood sugar. Microwaving oatmeal with an egg is a built-in solution in one bowl. Add more fiber-filled fruit and nuts for a burst of flavor and textures.

½ cup unsweetened almond milk or milk of choice
⅓ cup old-fashioned oats
1/16 teaspoon kosher salt
1 large egg

1 In a medium microwave-safe bowl, add milk, oats, and salt and stir. Microwave 1 minute 30 seconds and then stir again.

2 In a small bowl or cup, crack egg and whisk well. Add egg to warm oats and stir until well combined.

3 Microwave another 30–45 seconds and enjoy!

Apple Pie Breakfast Tacos

Tacos for breakfast? These sweet, creamy, crunchy, and salty tacos are a unique twist on a typically savory handheld dish. Have one for a perfect snack, or two for breakfast. You can also serve apples over reduced-fat/fat-free ricotta cheese or vanilla Greek yogurt. Add nuts for extra protein and crunch if desired.

1 small Gala or Fuji apple, peeled, cored, and diced

¾ teaspoon lemon juice

1 packet stevia, divided

¼ teaspoon plus ⅛ teaspoon ground cinnamon, divided

1 teaspoon whipped butter

½ cup low-fat cottage cheese

2 whole-grain hard corn taco shells

SERVES 1	
Per Serving:	
Calories	300
Fat	11g
Saturated Fat	4g
Cholesterol	15mg
Sodium	530mg
Carbohydrates	34g
Fiber	9g
Sugar	14g
Added Sugars	0g
Protein	15g

1. In a small bowl, combine apple, lemon juice, ½ stevia packet, and ¼ teaspoon cinnamon and toss to combine.
2. Melt butter in a medium sauté pan over medium heat. Add apple mixture and sauté approximately 10 minutes until apples are softened.
3. In a blender or food processor, place cottage cheese and remaining ½ stevia packet. Pulse until smooth.
4. Divide cottage cheese mixture between taco shells and top with cooked apples. Garnish with remaining ⅛ teaspoon cinnamon and serve.

Quinoa Berry Bowl

SERVES 4

Per Serving:

Calories	270
Fat	9g
Saturated Fat	0.5g
Cholesterol	0mg
Sodium	120mg
Carbohydrates	40g
Fiber	6g
Sugar	6g
Added Sugars	0g
Protein	7g

SINGLE SERVING QUICK TIP

Use this basic recipe to make four servings at once, then refrigerate any leftover quinoa and microwave single portions as needed, adding fruit after warming. Use cooked quinoa within 3 days. Try other berries, nuts, or spices such as ginger or nutmeg to vary this nutritious breakfast cereal. If you need a touch more sweetness, sprinkle with a bit of stevia, or drizzle on a small amount of maple syrup or honey.

Quinoa isn't only for dinner. It's a blank canvas to decorate with sweet or savory ingredients to suit your taste preferences. Cooking it with a mixture of unsweetened nut milk and water will boost calcium intake and give it a creaminess that pairs well with fruit and nuts for a warm, satisfying, plant-based breakfast.

1 cup quinoa

1 cup water

1 cup unsweetened almond milk

½ teaspoon vanilla extract

⅛ teaspoon salt

1 teaspoon ground cinnamon

¼ cup coarsely chopped walnuts

3 cups strawberries, sliced

1 Rinse quinoa in a fine-mesh sieve or coffee filter until water runs clear.
2 In a medium saucepan, add quinoa, water, milk, vanilla, and salt and bring to a boil over medium-high heat. Reduce heat to low, cover, and cook 15 minutes or until all liquid has been absorbed. Stir in cinnamon.
3 Meanwhile, toast walnuts on a small baking sheet in toaster oven for approximately 2½ minutes, taking care not to burn them.
4 Divide quinoa into four bowls, add strawberries and toasted walnuts, and serve.

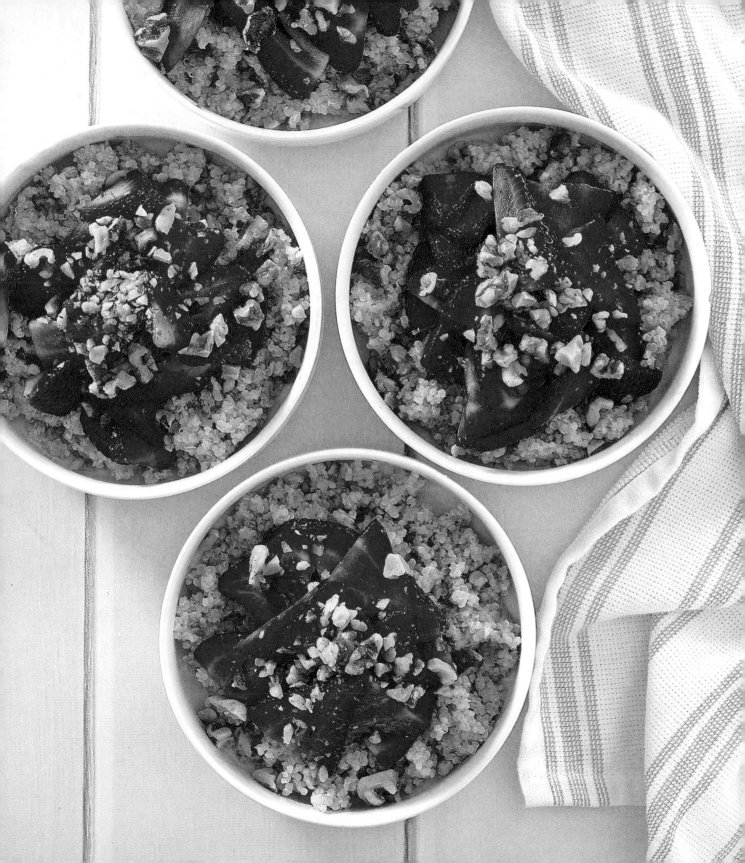

Blackberry Ricotta Breakfast Sorghum

Enjoy gluten-free, ancient grain goodness to start your day with this sweet, fiber-rich, hearty sorghum. Prep a batch in advance so all you need to do is serve it up in the morning. You can use either fresh or frozen blackberries for this dish. This recipe is also delicious with strawberries, blueberries, and raspberries.

SERVES 1

Per Serving:

Calories	300
Fat	8g
Saturated Fat	2.5g
Cholesterol	20mg
Sodium	320mg
Carbohydrates	50g
Fiber	9g
Sugar	8g
Added Sugars	0g
Protein	15g

ANCIENT GRAIN SORGHUM

Sorghum is a hearty ancient grain that's gluten free and rich in antioxidants and gut-healthy prebiotic fiber. Some sorghum varieties take longer to cook than others, so look for whole-grain sorghum that cooks in about 45 minutes on the stove or 15 minutes in a pressure cooker/Instant Pot®. This recipe can be served warm or cold.

¼ cup uncooked whole-grain sorghum

1 cup unsweetened vanilla almond or coconut milk

2 packets stevia, divided

¼ teaspoon ground cinnamon

¼ cup low-fat ricotta cheese

½ teaspoon lemon juice

¾ cup blackberries

Zest from ¼ medium lemon

1 In a medium pan, cook sorghum according to package directions using unsweetened milk instead of water. Once milk is mostly absorbed, remove from heat and let cool. Stir in 1 stevia packet and cinnamon. (To save time, prepare in a pressure cooker/Instant Pot® in about 15 minutes.)

2 In a medium bowl, combine ricotta, lemon juice, and another ½ stevia packet. Set aside.

3 In a small microwave-safe bowl, microwave blackberries 30–45 seconds until slightly juicy but still intact. Stir in remaining ½ stevia packet.

4 In a serving bowl, add sorghum and spread across bottom. Add ricotta mixture, then blackberries. Garnish with lemon zest. Serve.

Strawberry Vanilla Protein French Toast

This French toast recipe will help make your hectic mornings easy and nutritious. The secret to maximizing the protein content is to whisk Greek yogurt with the eggs instead of milk. Using fruit and yogurt as toppings adds sweetness and moisture. If you'd like you can top this off with a touch of maple syrup and cinnamon.

2 large eggs

1 (5.3-ounce) container low-sugar nonfat vanilla Greek yogurt, divided

½ teaspoon ground cinnamon

6 slices high-fiber, light wheat bread (40–50 calories per slice)

2 cups fresh strawberries, sliced

1 In a medium bowl, beat eggs. Whisk in ½ cup yogurt and cinnamon.

2 Spray a large sauté pan or griddle with nonstick cooking spray over medium to medium-high heat.

3 One at a time, dip both sides of bread into egg mixture and place in pan. Cook, flipping once, for about 3 minutes per side until lightly browned.

4 Transfer to a medium plate and cover to keep warm.

5 When ready to serve, stack three slices of French toast on each plate, and evenly top with remaining yogurt and strawberries.

SERVES 2	
Per Serving (3 slices):	
Calories	280
Fat	7g
Saturated Fat	1.5g
Cholesterol	190mg
Sodium	470mg
Carbohydrates	55g
Fiber	24g
Sugar	14g
Added Sugars	0g
Protein	19g

WHOLE EGGS ARE OKAY!

Don't toss those yolks! Yolks contain most of the egg's nutrients like vitamin D, vitamin B₁₂, selenium, and more than 40 percent of the protein. Eggs also include two important nutrients for brain health— choline and lutein. The US Dietary Guidelines removed cholesterol as a nutrient of concern so it's fine for most people to include whole eggs as part of a healthy diet in moderation.

Pumpkin Pie Smoothie

Per Serving:

Calories	220
Fat	3.5g
Saturated Fat	1g
Cholesterol	10mg
Sodium	460mg
Carbohydrates	30g
Fiber	5g
Sugar	17g
Added Sugars	0g
Protein	17g

CHOOSING A NUT MILK

Unsweetened almond milk can be used interchangeably with unsweetened coconut, cashew, soy, or oat milk in most recipes. Just check to make sure that there are no added sugars. Even "plain" varieties sometimes contain added sugar, so don't be tricked by the name. Always check the ingredient list and the "added sugars" line on the Nutrition Facts label.

Pumpkin is a fabulous source of many nutrients including vitamins A and C, potassium, zinc, and fiber. Keeping a can of pure pumpkin in your pantry means you can benefit from its many culinary uses all year round. Enjoy the flavors of pumpkin pie in this protein- and fiber-packed smoothie.

½ cup canned pure pumpkin

½ medium banana, preferably frozen

½ cup low-fat cottage cheese

½ cup unsweetened vanilla almond milk

1 teaspoon pumpkin pie spice, plus more for garnish

½ teaspoon vanilla extract

2 packets stevia

1 cup ice

Place all ingredients into a blender and process until desired consistency is achieved. Pour into a glass and dust with extra pumpkin pie spice as a garnish. Serve.

Cranberry Orange Protein Baked Oatmeal

Fresh cranberries are a fall gem to include in your favorite recipes, and they pair so well with citrus flavors. Grab one of these baked oatmeal pieces as a handheld breakfast, top it with some ricotta cheese, or crumble a piece on a Greek yogurt cup.

2 cups old-fashioned oats

1 teaspoon baking powder

1 teaspoon ground cinnamon

½ teaspoon salt

3½ packets stevia, divided

¼ cup ground flaxseed meal

½ cup vanilla plant-based protein powder

½ cup unsweetened vanilla almond milk

½ cup orange juice

1 teaspoon orange zest

½ cup nonfat plain Greek yogurt

3 tablespoons liquid egg whites

1 medium ripe banana, mashed

1 teaspoon vanilla extract

1 cup fresh cranberries, divided

SERVES 6	
Per Serving:	
Calories	220
Fat	4.5g
Saturated Fat	0g
Cholesterol	0mg
Sodium	330mg
Carbohydrates	34g
Fiber	5g
Sugar	8g
Added Sugars	0g
Protein	13g

1. Preheat oven to 350°F. Line a 9" × 9" brownie pan with parchment paper and set aside.
2. In a large bowl, combine oats, baking powder, cinnamon, salt, 3 packets stevia, and flaxseed and mix together. In a medium bowl, add all remaining ingredients except cranberries and ½ packet stevia and combine well.
3. Add wet ingredients to dry ingredients and gently combine. Stir in ½ cup of cranberries.
4. Pour mixture into pan and spread evenly. Top with remaining cranberries and gently press them into batter. Sprinkle them with remaining ½ packet stevia.
5. Bake 27–30 minutes or until toothpick inserted in middle comes out clean. Take care not to overcook it or the product will be dry. Let cool completely before slicing and serving. Cover and refrigerate leftovers for up to 5 days.

FRESH CRANBERRIES

Fresh cranberries are harvested in the fall and available in stores until early January—get them while you can (and buy some extra to freeze for later). Fresh cranberries are a versatile fruit that adds unique flavor, color, and variety to dishes—sweet or savory. They are a source of vitamin C and fiber, and naturally low in sugar. Cranberry products contain flavonoids and polyphenols, which are natural compounds that can support cardiovascular health.

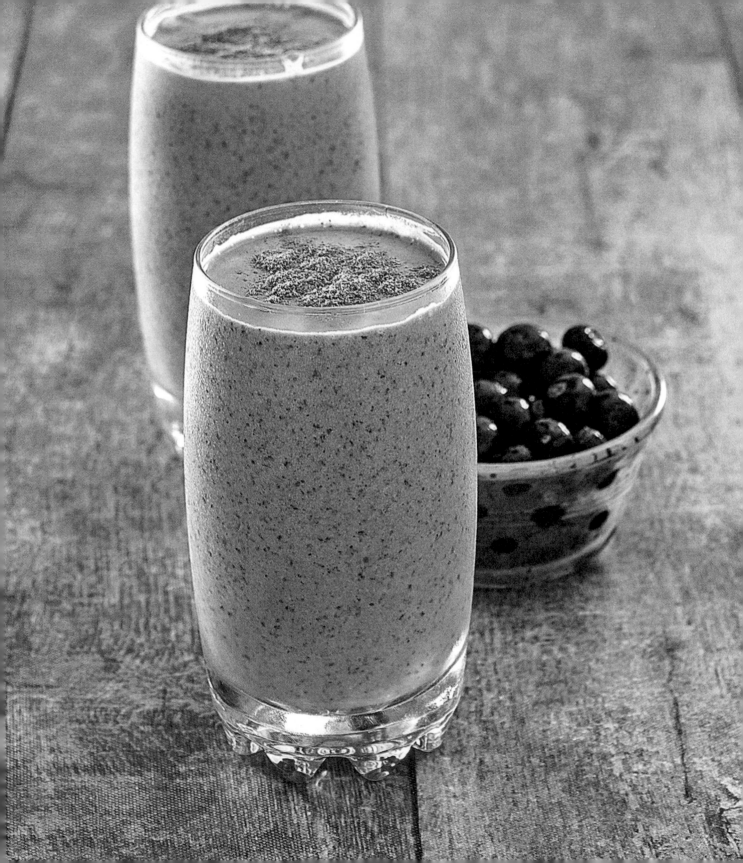

Wild Blueberry Peanutty Protein Smoothie

This antioxidant powerhouse smoothie is packed with plant-based protein thanks to its secret ingredient—tofu!

¾ cup unsweetened almond milk

¼ cup powdered peanut butter, plus more for garnish

4 ounces firm tofu, drained and patted dry

1 packet stevia

1 tablespoon ground flaxseed meal

1 cup frozen wild blueberries

½ cup ice cubes

1 Place all ingredients into a blender and process until smooth.

2 Pour into a tall glass and garnish with a sprinkle of extra powdered peanut butter. Serve.

SERVES 1

Per Serving:

Calories	330
Fat	12g
Saturated Fat	0g
Cholesterol	0mg
Sodium	320mg
Carbohydrates	36g
Fiber	13g
Sugar	12g
Added Sugars	0g
Protein	23g

WILD BLUEBERRY BENEFITS

Frozen wild blueberries (the tiny ones) contain twice as much antioxidant power as regular blueberries you find in the produce section. They also have been shown in studies to decrease insulin resistance, which helps control blood sugar with pre-diabetes.

Tomato and Feta Omelet

SERVES 1

Per Serving:

Calories	170
Fat	9g
Saturated Fat	4.5g
Cholesterol	205mg
Sodium	350mg
Carbohydrates	5g
Fiber	1g
Sugar	4g
Added Sugars	0g
Protein	16g

VEGETABLES FOR BREAKFAST

Omelets are a great low-carb breakfast and an easy way to include vegetables in your first meal of the day. This recipe comes together in only 10 minutes. Try using fresh herbs as a garnish instead of salt. If you do wish to add salt, try ⅛ teaspoon of kosher salt at the end so it will hit your palate right away and minimize the total amount you need.

A helpful omelet trick is to combine whole eggs and egg whites to maintain color and texture while managing the total fat and calories in your dish. Tomatoes and feta make a lovely flavor combo, and a garnish of fresh herbs adds brightness to any meal.

2 large egg whites (or ¼ cup liquid egg whites)

1 large whole egg

2 tablespoons crumbled feta cheese

½ cup chopped tomatoes

⅛ teaspoon ground black pepper

1 teaspoon chopped fresh cilantro or parsley

1 In a medium bowl, place egg whites and whole egg and whisk together.

2 Add feta, tomatoes, and pepper and stir to combine.

3 Spray a small skillet with nonstick cooking spray over medium heat. Add mixture and cook 4 minutes or until eggs are firm. Do not stir.

4 Flip and cook other side 2 additional minutes. Garnish with chopped fresh cilantro or parsley before serving.

Cheesy Flax Muffins

Muffins don't have to be sweet. These savory egg and cheese-based muffins are packed with protein, fiber, and heart-healthy omega-3 fats. Enjoy two with a side of berries for a very satisfying morning. If you can't find Pecorino-Romano cheese, Parmesan will work too.

⅔ cup reduced-fat (2%) cottage cheese

¼ cup grated Pecorino-Romano cheese

¼ cup white whole-wheat flour

⅔ cup ground flaxseed meal

1 teaspoon baking powder

3 large eggs

3 tablespoons water

½ cup shredded reduced-fat (2%) Mexican cheese

2 tablespoons chopped fresh chives

1 Preheat oven to 400°F. Spray eight muffin tin cups with nonstick cooking spray or add liners.

2 In a medium mixing bowl, combine cottage cheese, Pecorino-Romano, flour, flaxseed, baking powder, eggs, and water. Mix until well combined and then gently stir in shredded cheese and chives. Divide batter evenly into prepared muffin cups.

3 Bake 20 minutes or until lightly browned on top and set. Make sure to cool completely before removing liners to prevent sticking and serve.

SERVES 8	
Per Serving:	
Calories	130
Fat	8g
Saturated Fat	2.5g
Cholesterol	80mg
Sodium	230mg
Carbohydrates	5g
Fiber	2g
Sugar	1g
Added Sugars	0g
Protein	10g

Peanut Butter Banana Chia Pudding

SERVES 1

Per Serving:

Calories	310
Fat	16g
Saturated Fat	1.5g
Cholesterol	0mg
Sodium	380mg
Carbohydrates	32g
Fiber	17g
Sugar	7g
Added Sugars	0g
Protein	17g

WHY CHIA SEEDS?

Chia seeds are especially useful in weight management because they absorb up to ten times their weight in water, making them very filling. Switch up any combo of chia seeds, milk, fruit, and nuts to create many varieties of this easy, make-ahead breakfast.

This breakfast chia pudding is gluten-free and rich in plant-based protein, fiber, and heart-healthy fats thanks to powdered peanut butter and super-satisfying chia seeds. Just one serving provides 75 percent of daily fiber needs! If you don't like almond milk, unsweetened cashew, oat, or coconut milk can be substituted.

¼ medium ripe banana, mashed

2 tablespoons chia seeds

3 tablespoons powdered peanut butter

1 packet stevia

⅔ cup unsweetened almond milk

For garnish

3 slices banana

2 teaspoons powdered peanut butter mixed with water

1 teaspoon chopped peanuts (approximately 4 peanuts)

1 In a Mason jar or container with a lid add all ingredients except garnish and mix very well.
2 Cover and let sit in refrigerator overnight.
3 When ready to serve, stir pudding and top with banana slices, drizzle prepared peanut butter sauce on top, add chopped peanuts, and serve.

Blueberry Protein Pancakes

These deliciously simple pancakes are gluten-free, dairy-free, and made with no added sugar. Whip up a batch on the weekend to enjoy on busy weekday mornings.

½ cup old-fashioned oats

1 large egg

¼ cup plus 2 tablespoons liquid egg whites

1 medium ripe banana, mashed

¼ teaspoon vanilla extract

½ teaspoon baking powder

½ cup blueberries

1 In a blender or food processor, pulse oats until they are ground but not powdery.

2 In a medium bowl, beat egg and egg whites. Add oats, banana, vanilla, and baking powder, stirring to combine. Gently stir in blueberries.

3 Spray a large sauté pan or griddle with nonstick cooking spray over medium heat and use a ¼-cup measuring cup to scoop batter onto pan.

4 Cook bottom for 2–4 minutes until golden brown and then carefully flip over and cook another 2–4 minutes until set and golden. Serve warm.

SERVES 2

Per Serving (3 pancakes):

Calories	210
Fat	4.5g
Saturated Fat	1g
Cholesterol	95mg
Sodium	270mg
Carbohydrates	33g
Fiber	4g
Sugar	12g
Added Sugars	0g
Protein	12g

DOUBLE THE BATCH AND FREEZE

These pancakes are freezer friendly. Let pancakes cool completely, then wrap in parchment paper and place in a freezer-safe zip-top plastic bag. To reheat, try microwaving 30 seconds at a time, flipping as needed. Avoid overheating! Top with cottage cheese or low-fat ricotta cheese if desired to up the protein intake.

Pumpkin Chip Protein Mug Cake

TIPS

This mug cake works best with plant-based protein powder. Whey protein will yield a much tougher product—think hockey puck if it's over-cooked. It's okay if the top is a little moist or slightly undercooked. The recipe uses liquid egg whites, which are pasteurized so it's not necessary to make sure they are thoroughly cooked.

Pumpkin isn't just for pie. This protein- and fiber-packed mug cake has a "dessert for breakfast" kind of feel without the carbs and sugar you would expect in a cake. You can use coconut flour or another gluten-free flour in place of the almond flour.

¼ cup vanilla plant-based protein powder

¾ teaspoon pumpkin pie spice

½ teaspoon baking powder

1 packet stevia

2 tablespoons almond flour

3 tablespoons liquid egg whites

¼ cup canned pure pumpkin

2 tablespoons unsweetened almond milk

2 tablespoons unsweetened applesauce

2 teaspoons mini chocolate chips, divided

1   In a wide, microwave-safe flat-bottomed mug add protein powder, pumpkin pie spice, baking powder, stevia, and flour and whisk to combine.

2   Add egg whites, pumpkin, milk, and applesauce and whisk to thoroughly combine, making sure there is no powder left in the bottom of the mug. Stir in 1 teaspoon chocolate chips.

3   Microwave 2 minutes or until set without the top looking wet. Let sit in the microwave for 1–2 minutes to finish cooking and top with remaining 1 teaspoon chocolate chips. Serve immediately.

Banana Flax Muffin in a Mug

If you love muffins, you'll love the delicious taste and quick cooking of this one—it cooks in 2 minutes in the microwave! The flaxseed meal substitutes beautifully for the traditional flour and contributes fabulous amounts of fiber, plant-based protein, and omega-3 fats.

¼ cup ground flaxseed meal

¾ teaspoon baking powder

2 teaspoons ground cinnamon

1 packet stevia

3 tablespoons liquid egg whites (or 1 large whole egg)

1 teaspoon whipped butter

½ teaspoon vanilla extract

¼ medium ripe banana, chopped small but not mashed, plus 3 slices banana

2 tablespoons low-sugar, nonfat vanilla Greek yogurt, divided

1 In a large microwave-safe mug, add flaxseed meal, baking powder, cinnamon, and stevia and stir.

2 Add egg whites, butter, vanilla, chopped banana, and 1 tablespoon Greek yogurt. Combine well and cook in microwave 1½–2 minutes until firm.

3 Let stand for 1–2 minutes. Top with remaining 1 tablespoon yogurt and garnish with banana slices.

SERVES 1	
Per Serving:	
Calories	250
Fat	11g
Saturated Fat	1g
Cholesterol	5mg
Sodium	370mg
Carbohydrates	24g
Fiber	10g
Sugar	6g
Added Sugars	0g
Protein	14g

Avocado Toast with Turkey Bacon and Tomatoes

SERVES 1

Per Serving:

Calories	210
Fat	9g
Saturated Fat	1g
Cholesterol	40mg
Sodium	560mg
Carbohydrates	33g
Fiber	17g
Sugar	4g
Added Sugars	0g
Protein	15g

CHOOSING TURKEY BACON

There are many varieties of turkey bacon. Look for one with 5–6 grams of protein per slice and preferably lower in sodium. If possible, look for uncured as well, meaning it is made without sodium nitrate.

Move over BLT, these open-faced avocado toasts are creamy, crunchy, salty, and addictive. Subbing avocado for mayonnaise adds heart-healthy fat and fiber while keeping that smooth texture.

2 slices uncured turkey bacon

2 slices light, high-fiber wheat bread

¼ medium avocado, peeled, pitted, and sliced

1 small vine tomato, sliced

1⁄16 teaspoon ground black pepper

1 Place turkey bacon between two paper towels and microwave 2–2½ minutes until desired crispness is achieved.

2 Meanwhile, toast bread in toaster to desired doneness.

3 In a small bowl, mash avocado with a fork until smooth and spread on toast.

4 Break bacon slices in half and top toast with two halves each. Add tomato slices and sprinkle with black pepper. Serve.

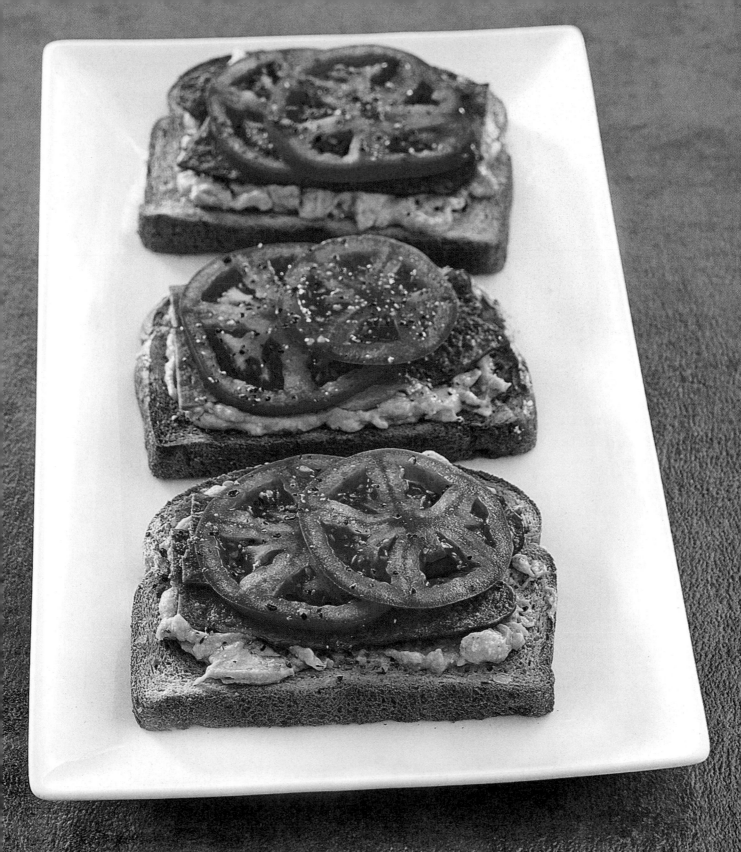

Peanut Butter Banana Protein Baked Oatmeal

SERVES 6

Per Serving:

Calories	200
Fat	3.5g
Saturated Fat	0g
Cholesterol	0mg
Sodium	380mg
Carbohydrates	31g
Fiber	4g
Sugar	6g
Added Sugars	0g
Protein	13g

BAKING WITH PROTEIN POWDER

Baking with protein powder helps to pump up the protein content of your breakfast. Whey protein is fine to use from a nutritional perspective, but it tends to toughen up baked goods. Plant-based (vegan) protein powders yield a more tender product. It's up to you which to choose, though you may want to cut a couple of minutes off the cooking time if using whey.

Baked oatmeal is a fabulous way to meal prep breakfast for the week. Eat it cold, warm, or topped with a dollop of Greek yogurt or cottage cheese for extra protein.

2 cups old-fashioned oats

1 teaspoon baking powder

1 teaspoon ground cinnamon

½ teaspoon salt

3 packets stevia

½ cup powdered peanut butter

¼ cup vanilla plant-based protein powder

1 cup unsweetened vanilla almond milk

½ cup nonfat plain Greek yogurt

3 tablespoons liquid egg whites

1 medium ripe banana, mashed

1 teaspoon vanilla extract

1 medium ripe banana, sliced in 24 slices

1 Preheat oven to 350°F. Line a 9" × 9" brownie pan with parchment paper.
2 In a large bowl, combine oats, baking powder, cinnamon, salt, stevia, powdered peanut butter, and protein powder.
3 In a separate large bowl, combine milk, yogurt, egg whites, mashed banana, and vanilla extract.
4 Slowly add oat mixture to wet ingredients and gently stir until fully combined.
5 Pour mixture into pan and spread it evenly. Top with banana slices (four rows of six slices each).
6 Bake 27–30 minutes or until golden brown and set. Let cool and cut into six rectangles. Wrap and refrigerate extras until ready to serve.

Fruity Egg Wraps

A cross between a crepe and an omelet, these high-protein, low-carb egg wraps can be a vessel for almost any filling, savory or sweet. Instead of the fruit spread called for here, you can also use the Blueberry Chia Jam recipe in this chapter. If you'd like you can top these with extra fruit spread before serving.

2 large eggs

¼ cup plus 2 tablespoons liquid egg whites

⅛ teaspoon kosher salt

1½ tablespoons low-sugar fruit spread

1 tablespoon chopped walnuts, toasted (about ¼ ounce)

1 Heat a medium sauté pan over medium to medium-high heat and spray with nonstick cooking spray.

2 In a small bowl, whisk eggs, egg whites, and salt together until frothy.

3 Pour about ¼ cup egg mixture into pan and tilt to create a thin layer. Cook 1–2 minutes until lightly browned on bottom, then gently flip to other side. Cook 1 minute more. When done, place egg wrap on a medium plate and repeat with remaining egg mixture to make two more wraps.

4 To serve, add 2 teaspoons fruit spread to each egg wrap, fold it up on both sides, and roll as if you are making a burrito to contain filling. Top with walnuts and serve.

SERVES 1	
Per Serving (3 wraps):	
Calories	260
Fat	15g
Saturated Fat	3.5g
Cholesterol	370mg
Sodium	530mg
Carbohydrates	9g
Fiber	1g
Sugar	0g
Added Sugars	0g
Protein	24g

Smoked Salmon Wrap

CHOOSING SMOKED SALMON

If smoked salmon is a staple for you, try to find a nitrate-free version. Also, this recipe is higher in sodium than most. If you have health issues requiring you to limit the sodium in your diet, only enjoy it once in a while.

If you are a fan of bagels with lox but not the 700 calories and 80 grams of carbs in a deli bagel sandwich, swapping it for a high-fiber wrap gives you the best of both worlds.

1 high-fiber, low-carb tortilla wrap (60–80 calories)
3 teaspoons light cream cheese, divided
2 ounces smoked salmon
1 small tomato, sliced
8 slices cucumber
¼ teaspoon everything bagel seasoning

1 On a medium plate, lay wrap flat and spread 2 teaspoons cream cheese along center from end to end. Add smoked salmon, tomato, and cucumber slices on top of cream cheese and sprinkle with everything seasoning.

2 Roll as tightly as possible to keep filling from falling out of wrap, then spread remaining 1 teaspoon cream cheese on exposed outer edge to help create a seal. Slice in half and serve.

Chocolate-Pomegranate Overnight Oats

Prep these oats at night and all you need in the morning is a spoon to enjoy this protein-packed, filling, blood sugar stabilizing, and guiltless way to indulge in chocolate for breakfast. You can substitute the whey with a plant-based protein powder if preferred. If almond milk isn't your thing, feel free to use unsweetened cashew, coconut, or oat milk.

⅓ cup old-fashioned oats

1 teaspoon chia seeds

1 tablespoon unsweetened cocoa powder

2 tablespoons chocolate whey protein powder

1 packet stevia

⅓ cup unsweetened vanilla almond milk

⅓ cup nonfat plain Greek yogurt

⅓ cup pomegranate arils, divided

1 In a Mason jar or container with a lid, add oats, chia, cocoa powder, protein powder, and stevia and stir.

2 Add milk and yogurt and stir again until no dry ingredients are visible.

3 Add pomegranate arils, reserving 1 tablespoon for garnish.

4 Cover and place in refrigerator several hours or overnight. When ready to eat, top with remaining 1 tablespoon pomegranate arils and enjoy.

SERVES 1	
Per Serving:	
Calories	280
Fat	6g
Saturated Fat	0g
Cholesterol	10mg
Sodium	130mg
Carbohydrates	38g
Fiber	8g
Sugar	11g
Added Sugars	0g
Protein	25g

THE BASICS OF OVERNIGHT OATS

If you have never tried overnight oats, they are life changing. The simple combination of old-fashioned oats, some form of milk (dairy or nondairy), and Greek yogurt is the base for an endless array of flavor combinations you can make at night and grab-and-go in the morning. If you prefer, you can heat it as well. You may add almost any topping while still benefitting from the filling and heart-healthy soluble fiber in the oats.

Asparagus and Artichoke Omelet Cups

Egg cups are an easy way to pack vegetables and protein into your breakfast. Serve with a side of berries for extra fiber. Meal prep these on Sunday to have breakfast ready to go for busy weekday mornings.

SERVES 9	
Per Serving:	
Calories	110
Fat	5g
Saturated Fat	2.5g
Cholesterol	50mg
Sodium	318mg
Carbohydrates	5g
Fiber	1g
Sugar	1g
Added Sugars	0g
Protein	9g

1 tablespoon olive oil

¼ cup chopped onion

¾ cup diced asparagus

1 (14-ounce) can artichoke hearts, rinsed, drained, and chopped

1 cup shredded reduced-fat (2%) Cheddar cheese

2 large eggs

½ cup liquid egg whites

½ cup low-fat cottage cheese

¼ teaspoon ground cayenne pepper

¼ teaspoon salt

⅛ teaspoon ground black pepper

1 Preheat oven to 375°F. Spray nine muffin tin cups generously with nonstick cooking spray.
2 In a large nonstick skillet over medium-high heat, heat olive oil. Add onion and sauté until translucent, about 5 minutes.
3 Add asparagus and artichoke hearts and cook an additional 3 minutes.
4 Divide cooked vegetables among prepared muffin cups. Sprinkle Cheddar on top.
5 In a small bowl, whisk eggs, egg whites, cottage cheese, cayenne, salt, and black pepper together and pour over vegetables.
6 Bake 16 minutes or until set and a toothpick inserted in center comes out clean.

High-Fiber Cereal–Crusted French Toast

Fiber up with the delightfully simple, whole-grain taste in this easy, sweet, soft, and crunchy French toast with a twist. Add your favorite fruit for an extra sweet morning.

1 large whole egg

1 large egg white

⅓ cup 1% milk

½ teaspoon ground cinnamon

½ teaspoon vanilla extract

1⁄16 teaspoon salt

⅔ cup high-fiber cereal, such as Fiber One

4 slices high-fiber, light whole-wheat bread (40–50 calories per slice)

1. In a medium wide, flat bowl, whisk together egg, egg white, milk, cinnamon, vanilla, and salt.
2. Add cereal to a zip-top plastic bag and crush with back of a spoon until you have small pieces, not dust. Pour onto a flat medium plate.
3. Spray a large sauté pan or griddle with nonstick cooking spray over medium-high heat.
4. Cut each bread slice diagonally so you have eight triangles. Dip each piece into egg mixture, coating both sides. Let excess drip off and then coat both sides with cereal.
5. Cook each piece on one side until browned and set, about 2 minutes. Flip and cook an additional 1–2 minutes. Serve immediately for best texture or reheat on foil in toaster oven to maintain crispness.

SERVES 2	
Per Serving:	
Calories	190
Fat	4.5g
Saturated Fat	1g
Cholesterol	95mg
Sodium	390mg
Carbohydrates	38g
Fiber	13g
Sugar	4g
Added Sugars	1g
Protein	13g

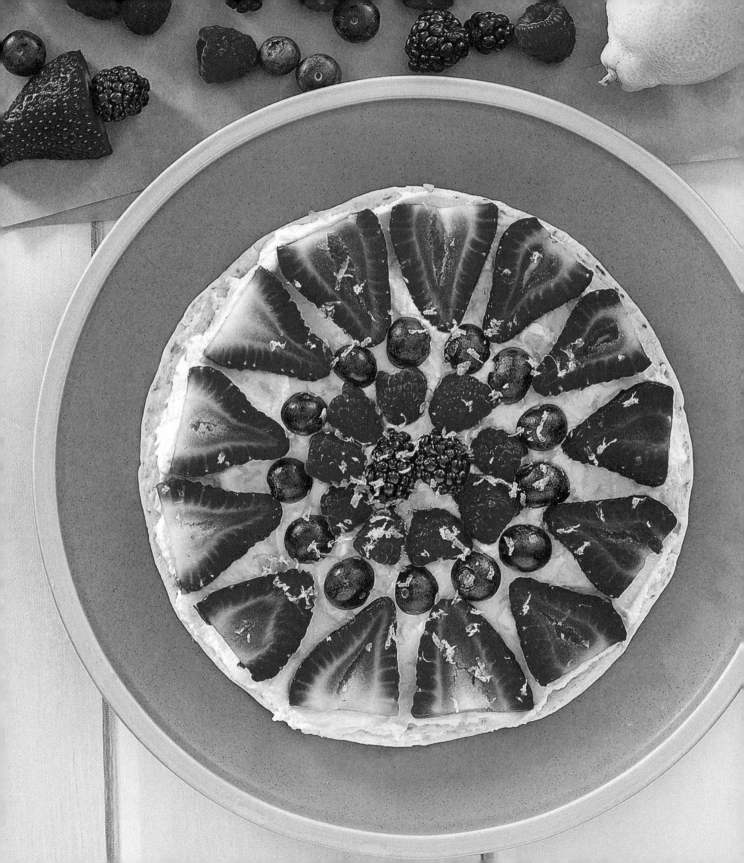

Berry Fruit Tart

This gorgeous creation is almost too beautiful to eat. A protein- and fiber-packed breakfast or dessert, it's bursting with heart-healthy benefits from berries and whole grains!

1 (8") high-fiber, low-carb flour tortilla

½ cup low-fat ricotta cheese

1 teaspoon lemon juice

1 teaspoon lemon zest, divided

2 packets stevia

4 medium strawberries, stemmed and thinly sliced

10 medium blueberries, halved

2 medium raspberries, halved

3 medium blackberries, halved

1 Preheat oven or toaster oven to 300°F. Line a large baking sheet with parchment paper. Place tortilla on sheet and spray with nonstick cooking spray. Bake 10 minutes or until crispy but not burned, and set aside.

2 In a small bowl, combine ricotta, lemon juice, ½ teaspoon lemon zest, and stevia. Spread ricotta mixture on baked tortilla.

3 Top ricotta mixture with fruit by arranging strawberries on outer edge, then a ring of blueberries inside strawberry circle. Place raspberries and blackberries in center.

4 Garnish with remaining ½ teaspoon lemon zest. Slice into six slices with a pizza cutter and serve.

SERVES 1

Per Serving:

Calories	220
Fat	8g
Saturated Fat	3g
Cholesterol	30mg
Sodium	460mg
Carbohydrates	40g
Fiber	19g
Sugar	16g
Added Sugars	0g
Protein	18g

HOW TO CHOOSE A TORTILLA

There are now many higher-fiber, lower-carbohydrate tortillas on the market. Look for ones that contain 60–100 calories and have a high percentage of fiber compared to the total grams of carbohydrate, with approximately 7–12 grams of fiber per tortilla. A good brand to try is Mission Carb Balance.

Tomato and Basil Egg Cups

These Mediterranean-inspired egg cups are surprisingly easy to make. Keep them in refrigerator up to 5 days, and reheat them in the microwave for a quick, fuss-free breakfast.

6 large eggs

½ cup liquid egg whites

3 tablespoons grated Parmesan cheese

¼ teaspoon kosher salt

⅛ teaspoon ground black pepper

1 cup halved cherry tomatoes

¼ cup chopped fresh basil

1 Preheat oven to 350°F. Spray a twelve-cup muffin tin with non-stick cooking spray.

2 In a large bowl, whisk eggs, egg whites, Parmesan, salt, and black pepper until light and fluffy. Stir in tomatoes and basil.

3 Divide mixture among prepared muffin cups and bake 22 minutes or until eggs are set, firm, and lightly browned. Serve warm or at room temperature.

Chocolate-Strawberry Protein Flatbread

Chocolate and strawberries make a delicious combo in this easy breakfast treat that tastes like dessert. Thanks to the powdered peanut butter, it's also packed with blood sugar stabilizing protein.

1 high-protein, high-fiber flatbread (about 100 calories)

3 tablespoons powdered peanut butter

1 tablespoon chocolate whey or plant-based protein powder

1 teaspoon cocoa powder

½ packet stevia

2–3 tablespoons water

6 medium strawberries, stemmed and sliced

1 Toast flatbread in a toaster 3 minutes or until lightly browned and crispy.

2 Meanwhile, in a small bowl, combine powdered peanut butter, protein powder, cocoa powder, stevia, and water. Stir until smooth and desired consistency is achieved; it should be thick but not too dry.

3 Spread peanut mixture onto warm flatbread and top with strawberries. Cut into slices and serve.

SERVES 1

Per Serving:	
Calories	240
Fat	4.5g
Saturated Fat	0g
Cholesterol	5mg
Sodium	390mg
Carbohydrates	42g
Fiber	16g
Sugar	9g
Added Sugars	0g
Protein	21g

STRAWBERRIES ARE NUTRITIONAL POWERHOUSES

Strawberries contain powerful antioxidants called anthocyanins and have been shown to improve insulin sensitivity in people with insulin resistance. That's great news for strawberry lovers.

Oat Crepes

SERVES 2

Per Serving (2 crepes):

Calories	120
Fat	2g
Saturated Fat	0.5g
Cholesterol	5mg
Sodium	80mg
Carbohydrates	17g
Fiber	2g
Sugar	4g
Added Sugars	0g
Protein	8g

A CREPE FOR ANY OCCASION

Crepes are a versatile base that can house sweet or savory fillings. Fill with cottage cheese or ricotta cheese and fresh fruit; chicken and tomato sauce; or sautéed spinach, mushrooms, and low-fat cheese for a delicious treat.

These three-ingredient crepes keep well in the refrigerator in a sealed container up to 3 days. Make a batch on the weekend and enjoy with your favorite filling any day of the week.

½ cup old-fashioned oats, ground into flour
¼ cup liquid egg whites
½ cup 1% milk

1 Place oat flour in a small bowl, form a well in the middle, and pour egg whites into well.
2 Add milk gradually while whisking briskly to form a smooth, thin batter. Let stand 5 minutes.
3 Spray a medium sauté pan generously with nonstick cooking spray over high heat 2 minutes until pan is very hot.
4 Pour a scant ¼ cup batter in a small circle in center of hot pan. Rock and swirl pan in a circular motion while holding it a few inches above heat to get batter to thinly coat pan. Put pan directly on burner.
5 Heat batter about 1 minute until edges start to curl up. Use a large spatula to flip crepe and heat another 45 seconds until very lightly browned. Take care not to burn them.
6 Place cooked crepe on a large plate and cover with a paper towel. Repeat cooking, spraying pan between each batch, to make three more crepes. (The crepes will begin to cook quicker as the pan gets hotter and may take as little as 30 seconds on each side.) Serve.

Lemon Tofu Crème

This gluten-free, sugar-free, plant-based, blended lemon tofu makes a delicious topping for breakfast foods, snacks, and desserts. Pair with your favorite fruit and nuts or seeds for a creamy, crunchy, filling meal.

8 ounces firm tofu, drained and patted dry

Zest and juice of 1 large lemon

4 packets stevia

2 cups strawberries, sliced

30 pistachios, shelled and chopped

1 In a small food processor or blender, add tofu, lemon zest and juice, and stevia. Blend until tofu is completely smooth.

2 Transfer to two small bowls and top with strawberries and pistachios. Serve.

SERVES 2	
Per Serving:	
Calories	200
Fat	9g
Saturated Fat	0.5g
Cholesterol	0mg
Sodium	60mg
Carbohydrates	20g
Fiber	6g
Sugar	8g
Added Sugars	0g
Protein	14g

Zucchini Home Fries

SERVES 7

Per Serving:

Calories	50
Fat	2g
Saturated Fat	0g
Cholesterol	0mg
Sodium	20mg
Carbohydrates	9g
Fiber	3g
Sugar	5g
Added Sugars	0g
Protein	3g

ADD VEGETABLES TO YOUR BREAKFAST

Pair this recipe with scrambled or poached eggs or fold it into an omelet as an easy way to incorporate vegetables into your morning meal.

Swap out potatoes for zucchini for a low-carb, low-calorie version of home fries. You'll be pleasantly surprised by how good they taste!

2 teaspoons olive oil, divided

1 medium red bell pepper, seeded and diced

1 medium green bell pepper, seeded and diced

½ cup diced white onion

4 medium zucchini, diced

½ teaspoon ground paprika

½ teaspoon chili powder

¼ teaspoon garlic powder

1 In a large skillet over medium-high heat, heat 1 teaspoon oil 30 seconds. Add bell peppers and onion and sauté 4 minutes until crisp-tender.

2 Add remaining 1 teaspoon oil, zucchini, paprika, chili powder, and garlic powder to skillet and sauté another 4 minutes until vegetables are lightly browned and slightly tender. Serve.

Scrambled Tofu with Mushrooms, Peppers, and Tomatoes

This plant-based alternative to scrambled eggs tastes surprisingly authentic for vegans and egg lovers alike. Turmeric is the key to the eggy color and also contains curcumin, which can help fight inflammation and potentially contributes to healthy blood sugar levels.

1 small onion, peeled and diced

1 medium clove garlic, peeled and minced

1 cup sliced mushrooms

1 small tomato, diced

1 small red bell pepper, seeded and diced

1 pound extra-firm tofu, drained

½ teaspoon all-purpose seasoning

½ teaspoon ground black pepper

½ teaspoon ground turmeric

1 Place a medium nonstick skillet over medium heat and coat with nonstick cooking spray. Add onion, garlic, mushrooms, tomato, and bell pepper and cook, stirring, 5 minutes.

2 Crumble tofu over top, keeping it in large chunks. Add all-purpose seasoning, black pepper, and turmeric and gently stir to combine. Cook another 5 minutes, stirring gently.

3 Remove from heat and serve immediately.

SERVES 4	
Per Serving:	
Calories	140
Fat	6g
Saturated Fat	0.5g
Cholesterol	0mg
Sodium	100mg
Carbohydrates	11g
Fiber	3g
Sugar	3g
Added Sugars	0g
Protein	14g

VERSATILE TOFU

Tofu soaks up flavors like nothing else and can be added to almost any type of dish, providing added protein, calcium, and iron. Cube a pound of extra-firm tofu, add assorted vegetables, and roast. Slice into sticks, bake, and toss with a little nutritional yeast. Crumble and add to a vegetable stir-fry with brown rice. Or use instead of chicken in a vegetarian noodle soup.

Cranberry Compote over Whole-Grain Waffles

SERVES 1

Per Serving:

Calories	310
Fat	9g
Saturated Fat	3g
Cholesterol	20mg
Sodium	730mg
Carbohydrates	46g
Fiber	6g
Sugar	11g
Added Sugars	2g
Protein	16g

HEALTH BENEFITS OF CRANBERRIES

Cranberries are rich in antioxidants called polyphenols, which have been shown to reduce diabetes risk and improve insulin sensitivity. Research has also shown that consuming cranberries may contribute to urinary tract health, gut health, and cardiovascular health.

The flavor combo of tart cranberries with lemon is like a party going on in your mouth. Piling it on top of creamy cottage cheese and whole-grain freezer waffles makes for quick, delicious comfort food.

1 cup fresh cranberries

1 teaspoon lemon juice

½ teaspoon lemon zest

1 packet stevia

2 whole-grain light frozen waffles

½ cup low-fat cottage cheese

1 Place cranberries in a medium microwave-safe bowl and cover loosely with a lid or paper plate to prevent splatter. Microwave on full power 2 minutes.

2 Add lemon juice, zest, and stevia and stir to combine.

3 Toast waffles to desired doneness.

4 Top waffles with cottage cheese and cranberry mixture and serve.

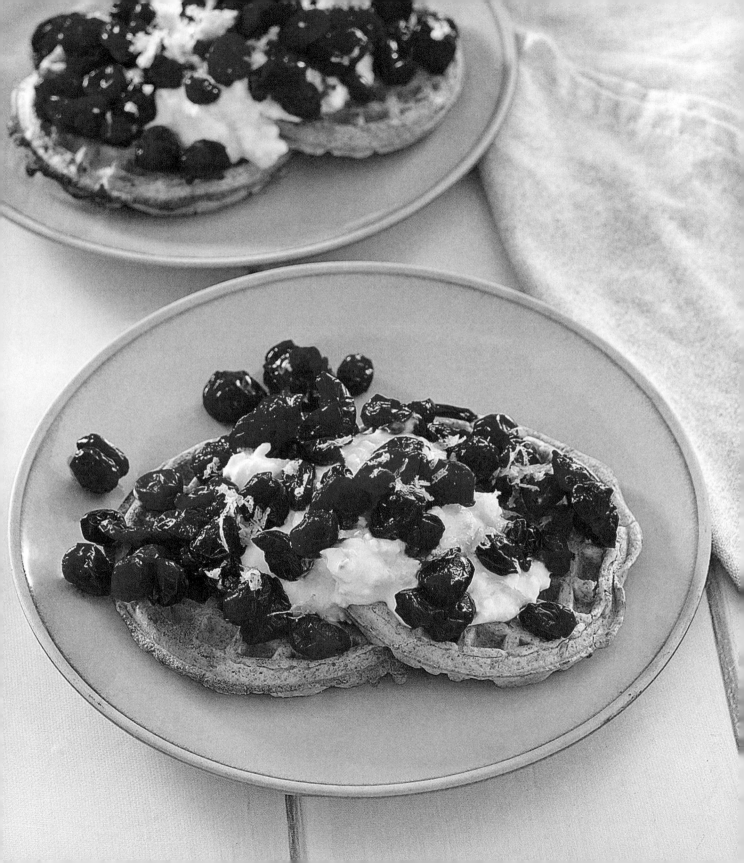

Asparagus, Swiss, and Ricotta Frittata

SERVES 4

Per Serving:

Calories	100
Fat	2.5g
Saturated Fat	1.5g
Cholesterol	10mg
Sodium	340mg
Fiber	1g
Sugar	4g
Added Sugars	0g
Protein	13g

Frittatas are impressive, yet ridiculously easy to make and an excellent way to incorporate an array of vegetables into breakfast. Use whichever combo you like, and if you do not have access to fresh vegetables, frozen or canned work just as well.

8 stalks asparagus, trimmed and cut into 1" pieces

1 medium shallot, peeled and finely diced

1¼ cups liquid egg replacement

¼ cup sliced jarred roasted red peppers

¼ cup shredded Swiss cheese

4 tablespoons low-fat ricotta cheese

1⁄16 teaspoon ground black pepper

1 Move rack to top of oven and preheat to 450°F.

2 Spray a medium ovenproof skillet with nonstick cooking spray over medium heat. Add asparagus and shallot and sauté 3 minutes. Add liquid egg replacement to skillet and remove from heat.

3 Top with red peppers and Swiss. Dollop 1 tablespoon ricotta over the top in each quarter of pan and season with black pepper.

4 Place skillet on top rack in oven and bake 10 minutes.

5 Remove from oven. Slide a heatproof spatula around and under frittata to loosen. Remove and cut into wedges. Serve immediately.

Carrot Cake Overnight Oats

The flavors and spices of carrot cake in a protein-rich breakfast makes for a true treat. And it's a terrific way to use up extra carrots, minimizing food waste.

⅓ cup old-fashioned oats

1 teaspoon chia seeds

2 tablespoons vanilla whey protein powder

1 packet stevia

½ teaspoon ground cinnamon

⅛ teaspoon ground allspice

¼ cup packed grated carrots

1 tablespoon raisins

⅓ cup unsweetened vanilla almond milk

⅓ cup plain nonfat Greek yogurt

½ teaspoon sugar-free maple syrup

1 tablespoon toasted and chopped walnuts

SERVES 1	
Per Serving:	
Calories	310
Fat	9g
Saturated Fat	1g
Cholesterol	10mg
Sodium	170mg
Carbohydrates	37g
Fiber	8g
Sugar	12g
Added Sugars	0g
Protein	24g

1 In a Mason jar or container with a lid, add all ingredients except walnuts and stir.
2 Top with walnuts.
3 Cover and refrigerate overnight. Serve.

Blueberry Chia Jam

MAKES ABOUT 1 CUP

Per Serving (1 tablespoon):

Calories	20
Fat	0.5g
Saturated Fat	0g
Cholesterol	0mg
Sodium	5mg
Carbohydrates	4g
Fiber	1g
Sugar	2g
Added Sugars	0g
Protein	1g

CHIA SEEDS

These amazing seeds are now easily found in stores. They absorb up to ten times their weight in water and contain fiber that can increase satiety and help to control blood sugar.

With no added sugar and tons of fiber, this jam is amazing as a crepe filling (see recipe in this chapter for Oat Crepes) or on oatmeal, cottage cheese, Greek yogurt, or a good ole PB and J sandwich. Substitute any fresh or frozen berries such as strawberries, raspberries, or blackberries. Increase the cooking time if the fruit is frozen.

2 cups blueberries

1 tablespoon lemon juice

2 tablespoons spoonable stevia

2 tablespoons chia seeds

1 In a loosely covered microwave-safe glass container, microwave blueberries on high power 2½ minutes. Smush any remaining whole blueberries with the back of a spoon.

2 Stir in lemon juice, stevia, and chia seeds. Place in refrigerator to thicken, about 20 minutes.

3 Enjoy immediately or store in an airtight container in refrigerator up to a week.

CHAPTER 3

Appetizers and Dips

Easy Onion Dip

Per Serving (2 tablespoons):	
Calories	35
Fat	2g
Saturated Fat	1.5g
Cholesterol	5mg
Sodium	20mg
Carbohydrates	1g
Fiber	0g
Sugar	1g
Added Sugars	0g
Protein	3g

Always a party staple, onion dip is usually very high in saturated fat. Subbing in Greek yogurt makes an everyday version to snack on with your favorite vegetables.

1 cup plain nonfat Greek yogurt

1 cup reduced-fat sour cream

2 tablespoons dried onion flakes

1 teaspoon kosher salt

¼ teaspoon lemon pepper

1 teaspoon dried dill

In a small bowl, mix all ingredients together. Cover and refrigerate 2–3 hours before serving.

Cilantro Peanut Pesto

Per Serving (2 tablespoons):	
Calories	70
Fat	6g
Saturated Fat	1.5g
Cholesterol	0mg
Sodium	75mg
Carbohydrates	4g
Fiber	1g
Sugar	1g
Added Sugars	0g
Protein	3g

A flavorful change from standard basil pesto, this zesty, Asian-inspired sauce is great on grilled seafood, chicken, steak, grains, pasta, wraps, and more.

½ cup fresh cilantro

¼ cup canned light unsweetened coconut milk

¼ cup unsalted peanuts

4 medium cloves garlic, peeled

Zest and juice of 1 medium lime

¼ teaspoon kosher salt

1 Place all ingredients into a food processor. Pulse until smooth.
2 Use immediately or store in an airtight container and refrigerate up to 5 days.

Fresh Baja Guacamole

Avocados act as nutrient boosters by helping increase the absorption of fat-soluble nutrients like vitamins A, D, K, and E. That means that dipping vegetables in this delicious guacamole will help you absorb even more of these important vitamins. Win-win! If you are sensitive to spicy foods, feel free to omit the serrano chili.

2 medium ripe avocados, peeled, pitted, and halved

½ cup minced red onion

2 tablespoons finely chopped fresh cilantro leaves

2 tablespoons lime juice

½ teaspoon kosher salt

¼ teaspoon ground black pepper

1 medium serrano chili, minced

½ medium tomato, chopped

1 Using a fork, mash avocados in a small bowl. Add onion, cilantro, lime juice, salt, black pepper, and serrano chili and mix together.

2 Stir in tomatoes just before serving.

SERVES 4	
Per Serving:	
Calories	130
Fat	11g
Saturated Fat	1.5g
Cholesterol	0mg
Sodium	150mg
Carbohydrates	9g
Fiber	5g
Sugar	2g
Added Sugars	0g
Protein	2g

WORKING WITH HOT CHILIES

Put on rubber gloves when handling hot chili peppers. They can sting, burn, and irritate the skin. Avoid touching your eyes during or after working with chilies. Be sure to wash your hands with soap and warm water right after. A good substitute for those who don't wish to handle a fresh hot pepper is jarred sliced jalapeños, which are even available in a "tamed" variety with a milder flavor.

Artichoke Spread

MAKES 1 CUP

Per Serving (2 tablespoons):	
Calories	50
Fat	2.5g
Saturated Fat	0.5g
Cholesterol	0mg
Sodium	250mg
Carbohydrates	4g
Fiber	1g
Sugar	1g
Added Sugars	0g
Protein	2g

Canned artichokes are a gift to add to dips and salads. They are one of the higher-fiber vegetables and add really interesting flavor to this hearty spread. Serve some with whole-grain crackers or spread on cucumbers, celery, or mini peppers. For a variation on this recipe, you can use sun-dried tomatoes instead of red peppers.

1 (14-ounce) can artichoke hearts, rinsed, drained, and patted dry

1 tablespoon chopped red onion

1 tablespoon chopped jarred roasted red pepper

1 tablespoon light mayonnaise

1 tablespoon reduced-fat sour cream

2 teaspoons grated Parmesan cheese

1 teaspoon lemon juice

½ teaspoon minced garlic

1 tablespoon olive oil

⅛ teaspoon ground black pepper

1 Place all ingredients into a food processor. Blend until smooth.

2 Refrigerate at least 3 hours before serving.

Garlic and Feta Cheese Spread

Feta and garlic are excellent partners and make for a tasty flavorful spread. Try it on cucumbers, stuffed into halved mini bell peppers, or inside hollowed cherry tomatoes.

½ cup crumbled feta cheese

4 ounces cream cheese, softened

¼ cup plain nonfat Greek yogurt

2 teaspoons roasted garlic paste

¼ teaspoon dried basil

¼ teaspoon dried oregano

⅛ teaspoon dried dill

⅛ teaspoon dried thyme

1 Place all ingredients into a food processor. Process until thoroughly mixed.

2 Cover and chill until ready to serve.

MAKES 1 CUP	
Per Serving (1 tablespoon):	
Calories	40
Fat	3.5g
Saturated Fat	2g
Cholesterol	10mg
Sodium	85mg
Carbohydrates	1g
Fiber	0g
Sugar	1g
Added Sugars	0g
Protein	1g

DRY-ROASTED GARLIC

Here's how you can make your own roasted garlic: Preheat oven to 350°F; lightly spray a covered baking dish with nonstick cooking spray. Slice off ½" from the top of a garlic head; rub off any loose skins, being careful not to separate cloves. Place in a baking dish, cut side up. Cover and bake until the garlic cloves are very tender when pierced, about 30–45 minutes. Will keep in the refrigerator 2–3 days.

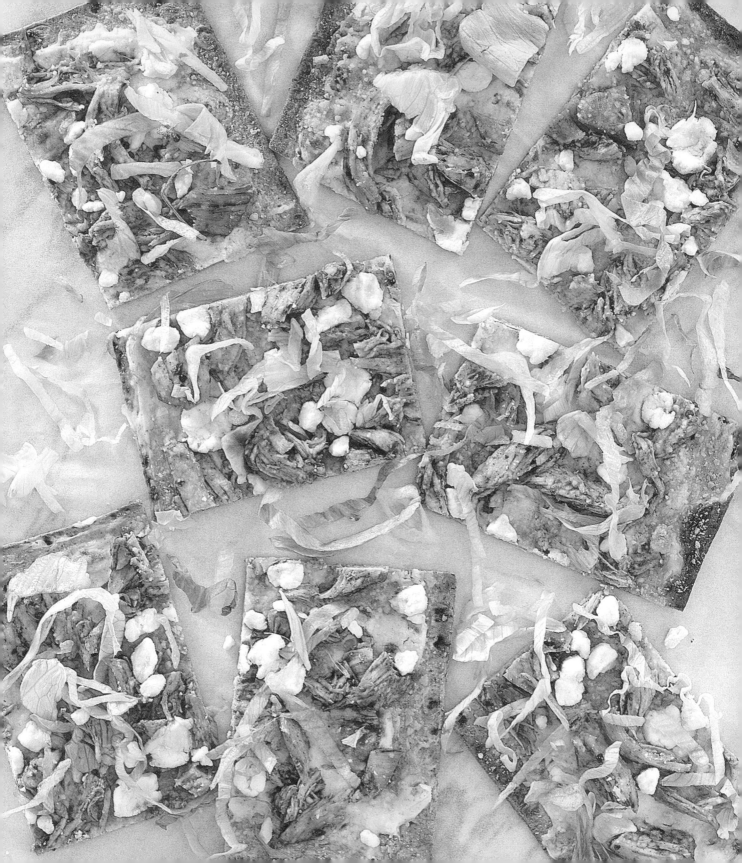

Buffalo Chicken Flatbread

Cheer on your team with a healthier version of this sports bar favorite finger food. Share or keep it all for yourself as a protein- and fiber-packed lunch or dinner.

1½ tablespoons light cream cheese

1 high-protein, high-fiber flatbread (about 100 calories)

3 ounces grilled or rotisserie chicken, shredded

1 tablespoon buffalo hot sauce

2 tablespoons loosely packed crumbled goat cheese

1 tablespoon grated Parmesan cheese

¼ cup shredded romaine lettuce

1 Preheat oven to 400°F.

2 Spread cream cheese evenly on flatbread.

3 In a small bowl, combine chicken and hot sauce. Distribute chicken evenly on flatbread.

4 Sprinkle with goat cheese and then Parmesan.

5 Bake directly on rack until cheese is slightly melted and flatbread is golden brown, approximately 5–8 minutes. Take care not to burn flatbread.

6 Top with shredded lettuce, cut into slices, and serve.

SERVES 1	
Per Serving:	
Calories	330
Fat	13g
Saturated Fat	7g
Cholesterol	110mg
Sodium	1,210mg
Carbohydrates	24g
Fiber	10g
Sugar	2g
Added Sugars	0g
Protein	40g

SODIUM WARNING

The sodium content of this recipe is fairly high at 1,210mg, but considering that hot wings served in a restaurant can contain 4,000–5,000mg of sodium per serving (upward of 500mg each wing), this dish will satisfy your cravings and serve as a much healthier alternative.

Cucumber Slices with Smoked Salmon Cream

Smoked salmon and cream cheese are a perfect pair. Serve this attractive low-carb appetizer to party guests and add the leftovers to a high-fiber wrap for a quick breakfast or lunch.

SERVES 8

Per Serving (3 pieces; 1 tablespoon cream cheese mixture):

Calories	45
Fat	3g
Saturated Fats	2g
Cholesterol	10mg
Sodium	140mg
Carbohydrates	2g
Fiber	1g
Sugar	1g
Added Sugars	0g
Protein	2g

MAKE IT FANCY

If you want to serve this as a fancy party dish, fit a pastry bag with a tip; spoon salmon cream into the bag and pipe 1 teaspoon atop each cucumber slice. If you do not have a pastry bag, use a plastic zip-top plastic bag and cut off one corner to squeeze out the cream cheese mixture. Don't have everything bagel seasoning? You can sprinkle the tops with additional dill and black pepper.

1 large seedless English cucumber, cut into ¼" diagonal slices (about 24 slices)

1 ounce smoked salmon

4 ounces ⅓ less fat cream cheese, softened

1 teaspoon lemon juice

¼ teaspoon ground black pepper

¼ teaspoon dried dill

1 teaspoon everything bagel seasoning

1 Place cucumbers on paper towels to drain while you prepare salmon cream.

2 In a food processor, combine salmon, cream cheese, lemon juice, black pepper, and dill. Blend until smooth.

3 Spread about 1 teaspoon salmon mixture on each cucumber slice. Garnish with bagel seasoning.

Spicy Southwest Sardine Bites

If you have never tried sardines or think you are not a fan, this tasty bite will blow your mind. Today's sardines are meaty and delicious, and the combo of salt, acid, and heat is a party in your mouth.

1 whole-grain flatbread (about 100 calories), cut into 10 pieces

⅛ teaspoon kosher salt

1 (4.25-ounce) package water-packed sardines, drained

Juice of 1 small lime

½ medium ripe avocado, peeled, pitted, and cut into 10 thin slices

20 jarred jalapeño pepper slices (about ⅓ cup)

¼ cup chopped fresh cilantro

2 teaspoons sriracha

1 Preheat oven or toaster oven to 350°F. Line a medium baking sheet with foil.

2 Place flatbread pieces on prepared baking sheet. Spray flatbread with olive oil spray and sprinkle with salt.

3 Bake about 8 minutes until flatbread pieces are lightly browned. Remove from oven and cool on a wire rack 2 minutes.

4 In a small bowl, place sardines and lime juice and gently stir to combine.

5 On each flatbread piece, stack 1 slice avocado, a small piece sardine, 2 jalapeño slices, a sprinkle of cilantro, and a drizzle of sriracha. Serve.

SERVES 10	
Per Serving:	
Calories	35
Fat	2g
Saturated Fat	0g
Cholesterol	5mg
Sodium	130mg
Carbohydrates	3g
Fiber	2g
Sugar	0g
Added Sugars	0g
Protein	3g

SUPER SARDINES

Sardines are a nutrition powerhouse as a low-mercury source of heart-healthy omega-3 fats. Shelf stable and affordable, they make a fabulous addition to your pantry.

Avocado, Black Bean, and Tomato Salad

SERVES 4

Per Serving:

Calories	190
Fat	11g
Saturated Fat	1.5g
Cholesterol	0mg
Sodium	270mg
Carbohydrates	23g
Fiber	10g
Sugar	2g
Added Sugars	0g
Protein	6g

NEED HELP RIPENING AVOCADOS FASTER?

Speed up the avocado ripening process by placing avocados in a paper bag with a kiwifruit or apple (or both). Apples, kiwifruit, and avocados all produce ethylene, which is a natural plant hormone that triggers the ripening process and is used commercially to help ripen bananas, avocados, and other fruit.

Classic game day party fare, this fiber-packed dish is healthy and delicious. Serve it as a dip with vegetables and high-fiber crackers or on top of a protein like grilled chicken or burgers.

1 large clove garlic, peeled and minced

½ small red onion, peeled and chopped

½ teaspoon kosher salt

½ teaspoon ground black pepper

3 tablespoons lime juice (from 1 large lime)

1 teaspoon sriracha

2 medium ripe avocados, peeled, pitted, and cut into cubes

1 cup halved grape tomatoes

1 cup canned low-sodium black beans, drained and rinsed

1 In a medium bowl, place garlic, onion, salt, black pepper, lime juice, and sriracha and stir to combine.

2 Gently fold in avocado, tomatoes, and beans and serve immediately or cover and refrigerate if you prefer to make it ahead of time.

Cheesy Dried Plum Flatbread

Cooking with dried plums is an easy way to add potassium, vitamin A, fiber, iron, and antioxidants to your meals. Research shows they also may help to strengthen bones and prevent or even reverse bone loss. This calorie-friendly flatbread is a fun appetizer to share or a sweet, creamy, salty meatless entrée for one.

¾ teaspoon extra-virgin olive oil

½ small red onion, peeled and thinly sliced

¼ cup low-fat cottage cheese

1 whole-grain, high-protein, and high-fiber flatbread (about 100 calories)

4 medium dried plums, diced

2 tablespoons crumbled goat cheese

1 teaspoon balsamic vinegar

SERVES 1	
Per Serving:	
Calories	330
Fat	10g
Saturated Fat	3.5g
Cholesterol	25mg
Sodium	480mg
Carbohydrates	54g
Fiber	14g
Sugar	21g
Added Sugars	0g
Protein	17g

1 Preheat oven to 400°F.

2 In a small sauté pan over medium heat, heat oil. Add onion and sauté until softened, about 10 minutes.

3 Spread cottage cheese on flatbread. Top with onion mixture and plums. Sprinkle with goat cheese.

4 Place flatbread directly on oven rack and bake until cheese is partially melted and starting to bubble. Drizzle with vinegar, slice, and serve.

Baked Coconut Shrimp

Per Serving (4 shrimp):

Calories	140
Fat	6g
Saturated Fat	4g
Cholesterol	105mg
Sodium	140mg
Carbohydrates	5g
Fiber	1g
Sugar	3g
Added Sugars	2g
Protein	16g

A lightened-up version of the deep-fried original, this crispy shrimp dish makes a fabulous party starter.

¼ cup almond flour

¼ rounded teaspoon ground cayenne pepper

¼ teaspoon kosher salt

2 teaspoons lime juice

2 teaspoons honey

¼ cup liquid egg whites

½ cup unsweetened shredded coconut

1 pound (about 24) extra-large shrimp, shelled with tails remaining and deveined

1 Preheat oven to 425°F. Spray a medium baking sheet with non-stick cooking spray and set aside.

2 In a small bowl, combine flour, cayenne, and salt.

3 In a separate small bowl, mix lime juice and honey. While continuously stirring, add egg whites to honey mixture.

4 Place coconut in a thin layer on a large flat dish. Dip each shrimp first into flour mixture, then into egg white mixture, and then roll in coconut.

5 Place on baking sheet. Spray tops with nonstick cooking spray and bake 10–15 minutes or until coconut appears lightly toasted. Serve.

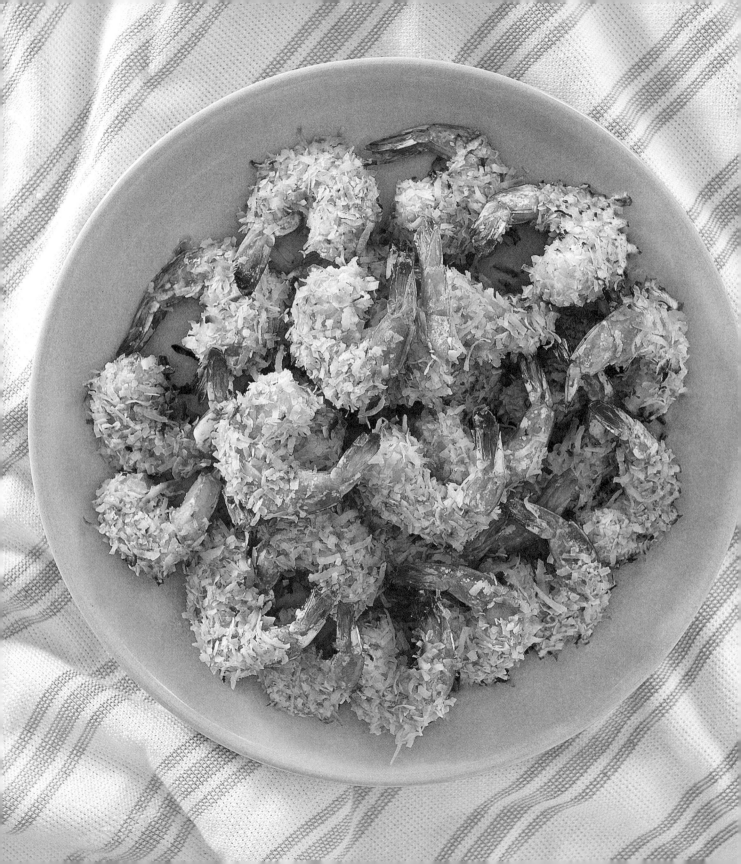

Three-Bean Avocado Salad with Lime Dressing

SERVES 16

Per Serving (½ cup):

Calories	130
Fat	6g
Saturated Fat	1g
Cholesterol	0mg
Sodium	150mg
Carbohydrates	16g
Fiber	6g
Sugar	3g
Added Sugars	0g
Protein	4g

Made almost entirely from pantry staples, this plant-based protein- and fiber-packed appetizer pairs well with everything from vegetables to burgers to stuffing for roasted squash.

1 (15-ounce) can low-sodium chickpeas, drained and rinsed

1 (15-ounce) can low-sodium black beans, drained and rinsed

1 (15-ounce) can low-sodium kidney beans, drained and rinsed

1 (15-ounce) can corn kernels, drained and rinsed

1 cup halved grape tomatoes

1 medium red bell pepper, seeded and diced

1 medium avocado, peeled, pitted, and diced

Juice of 1 large lime (about 3 tablespoons)

¼ cup extra-virgin olive oil

2 large cloves garlic, peeled and finely chopped

½ teaspoon kosher salt

¼ teaspoon ground black pepper

1 cup plus 1 tablespoon chopped fresh cilantro, divided

1 In a large mixing bowl, add beans, corn, tomatoes, and bell pepper.

2 In a small bowl, add avocado and lime juice, stirring to coat well to prevent browning. Using a slotted spoon, remove avocado from lime juice and add to bean mixture.

3 To the lime juice, add oil, garlic, salt, and black pepper, mix well, and pour over the salad, folding gently to combine.

4 Gently stir in 1 cup cilantro, cover, and refrigerate at least 1 hour to let the flavors develop.

5 Garnish with remaining 1 tablespoon cilantro before serving.

Black Bean Dip

Keep this dip with a kick in the refrigerator for snacking on vegetables or to add to salads, wraps, or even as a topping for a baked potato.

1 (15-ounce) can low-sodium black beans, drained and rinsed

½ cup diced yellow onion

4 medium cloves garlic, peeled and minced

2 teaspoons red hot pepper sauce

Juice of 1 medium lime (about 2 tablespoons)

½ cup reduced-fat sour cream

½ cup chopped fresh cilantro

½ teaspoon kosher salt

Place all ingredients into a food processor or blender. Pulse until smooth. Serve chilled or at room temperature.

Per Serving (2 tablespoons):	
Calories	40
Fat	1g
Saturated Fat	0.5g
Cholesterol	5mg
Sodium	90mg
Carbohydrates	5g
Fiber	2g
Sugar	0g
Added Sugars	0g
Protein	2g

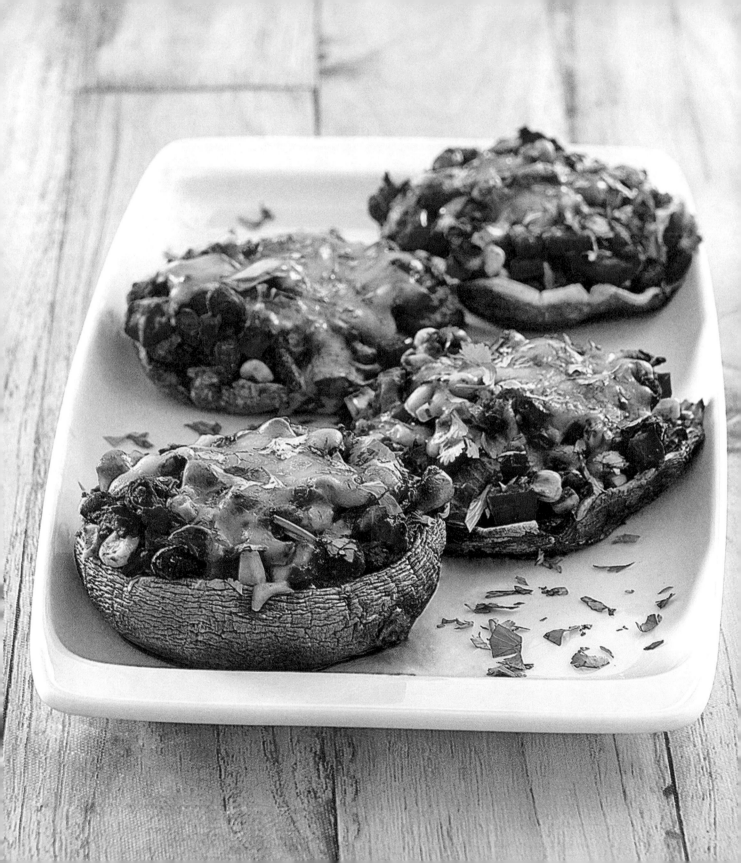

Portobello Mexican Pizzas

Using large portobello mushrooms instead of pizza crusts cuts the carbohydrates and increases the fiber in these tasty pizzas.

6 large portobello mushrooms (about 4"–5" in diameter), stemmed

1 teaspoon olive oil

1 cup diced white onion

2 cups chopped red bell pepper

1 (15-ounce) can low-sodium black beans, drained and rinsed

1 cup corn kernels, drained and rinsed

½ cup canned diced tomatoes, including juice

1 tablespoon ground cumin

2 teaspoons chili powder

¼ teaspoon garlic powder

¾ cup shredded reduced-fat (2%) Cheddar cheese

2 tablespoons chopped fresh cilantro

SERVES 6	
Per Serving:	
Calories	170
Fat	4.5g
Saturated Fat	2g
Cholesterol	10mg
Sodium	330mg
Carbohydrates	25g
Fiber	8g
Sugar	7g
Added Sugars	0g
Protein	11g

1 Preheat oven to 350°F. Spray a large baking sheet with nonstick cooking spray and set aside.

2 Place mushrooms on prepared baking sheet, stemmed side up. Bake 8 minutes.

3 While mushrooms are baking, heat oil in a medium skillet over medium heat 30 seconds.

4 Add onion and bell pepper and sauté 5 minutes until lightly browned and tender. Add beans, corn, tomatoes with juice, cumin, chili powder, and garlic powder and heat another 6 minutes, stirring occasionally. Set aside.

5 Remove mushrooms from oven and drain any excess moisture.

6 Return to baking sheet and stuff each mushroom with ½ cup filling.

7 Bake filled mushrooms 15 minutes. Remove from oven, sprinkle each with 2 tablespoons cheese, and bake another 2 minutes until cheese is slightly melted. Garnish with cilantro and serve.

Savory Stuffed Mushrooms

A lovely appetizer or light nosh, these stuffed mushrooms have a crisp and tasty breading that's so good, they'll be gone before you know it. This dish is great with white button or baby bella mushrooms.

1 pound fresh mushrooms, stems removed and reserved

2 tablespoons olive oil

½ cup Homemade High-Fiber Bread Crumbs (see Chapter 9)

1 large egg white

½ cup shredded Swiss cheese

4 medium cloves garlic, peeled

1 teaspoon dried Italian seasoning

¼ teaspoon kosher salt

½ teaspoon ground black pepper

1   Preheat oven to 400°F. Spray a medium baking sheet lightly with nonstick cooking spray and set aside.

2   Place mushroom stems into a food processor and add remaining ingredients except for mushroom caps. Pulse several times to finely chop and combine the mixture.

3   Stuff each mushroom cap with mixture, then place on prepared baking sheet. Place pan on middle rack in oven and bake 15 minutes. Mushrooms can be served warm or at room temperature.

Zucchini Sticks

Everything tastes good coated in breading, and these zucchini sticks are no exception. Make your own high-fiber bread crumbs to keep on hand to save money, carbs, and calories.

2 medium zucchini

1 large egg

1 tablespoon water

3 tablespoons Homemade High-Fiber Bread Crumbs (see Chapter 9)

1 tablespoon grated Parmesan cheese

1 teaspoon dried Italian seasoning

½ teaspoon garlic powder

½ teaspoon onion powder

¼ teaspoon ground black pepper

⅛ teaspoon ground sweet paprika

½ cup low-sodium marinara sauce

SERVES 4	
Per Serving:	
Calories	70
Fat	2.5g
Saturated Fat	1g
Cholesterol	50mg
Sodium	85mg
Carbohydrates	10g
Fiber	3g
Sugar	5g
Added Sugars	1g
Protein	5g

1 Preheat oven to 450°F. Spray a medium baking sheet with non-stick cooking spray and set aside.

2 Trim ends off zucchini, then cut in half. Quarter each of these halves, to make sixteen equal wedges.

3 In a small, shallow bowl, beat egg and water. Set aside.

4 In a small bowl, place Homemade High-Fiber Bread Crumbs, Parmesan, and seasonings and mix well to combine.

5 Dip each piece of zucchini in egg, then roll in bread crumbs mixture. Place on baking sheet and spray zucchini with nonstick cooking spray. Place baking sheet on middle rack in oven and bake 15 minutes. While zucchini is baking, gently warm pasta sauce on stovetop or in microwave. Pour into a small bowl and set aside.

6 Remove zucchini sticks from oven and serve immediately with warm sauce.

Mexican-Style Cucumber Boats

SERVES 6

Per Serving:

Calories	50
Fat	1g
Saturated Fat	0g
Cholesterol	0mg
Sodium	120mg
Carbohydrates	8g
Fiber	3g
Sugar	3g
Added Sugars	0g
Protein	3g

THE APPEAL OF PERSIAN CUCUMBERS

Persian cucumbers grow to only about 5"–6" long, have thin skins, and are very crunchy and mostly seedless. Low in calories, these cucumbers add crunch and fresh taste to salads. For a flavorful snack, sprinkle spears or slices with chili powder or a salt-free seasoning blend.

Scooped-out cucumber halves make a fun (and low-carb) vessel for ingredients commonly used in burritos. Not only are cucumber boats an attractive side dish, but they're also great for party appetizers or afternoon snacks. Two or three of them would even make a quick lunch.

6 tablespoons Black Bean Dip (see recipe in this chapter), or jarred black bean dip

3 medium Persian cucumbers, halved lengthwise and seeded

2 tablespoons canned corn kernels, drained and rinsed

2 tablespoons finely diced tomato

2 tablespoons chopped black olives

2 tablespoons shredded reduced-fat (2%) Cheddar cheese

1 Spread 1 tablespoon Black Bean Dip into depression of each cucumber half. Top with 1 teaspoon each corn, tomato, and olives.

2 Sprinkle each cucumber boat with 1 teaspoon cheese and serve immediately.

Walnut Pesto Sauce

Toasted walnuts bring the flavor to this versatile pesto. Keep a batch on hand to add to pasta, sandwiches, tortilla pizza, and so much more. This pesto can be stored in the refrigerator up to 5 days.

2 cups tightly packed fresh basil leaves

1½ ounces toasted walnuts (about rounded ⅓ cup)

¼ cup grated Parmesan cheese

1½ large cloves garlic, peeled and chopped

⅛ teaspoon salt

⅛ teaspoon ground black pepper

4 tablespoons extra-virgin olive oil, divided

1 Fill a medium saucepan halfway with water. Place over medium heat; bring to a boil. Next to saucepan, place a large bowl filled with water and ice. Drop a few basil leaves into boiling water. Blanch 3 seconds; quickly remove from boiling water with a slotted spoon and place in ice water. Repeat process until all basil has been blanched, adding ice to water as needed. Drain basil in colander and pat dry with a towel.

2 In a blender or food processor, combine walnuts, basil, Parmesan, garlic, salt, black pepper, and 3 tablespoons olive oil. Process until smooth and uniform.

3 Pour into airtight container and add remaining 1 tablespoon olive oil on top to act as protective barrier. Mix oil layer into pesto before using.

MAKES ABOUT 1 CUP	
Per Serving (1 tablespoon):	
Calories	60
Fat	6g
Saturated Fat	1g
Cholesterol	0mg
Sodium	45mg
Carbohydrates	1g
Fiber	0g
Sugar	0g
Added Sugars	0g
Protein	1g

TIPS

Blanching the basil will lend a bright green color to the pesto. If you are in a hurry, or plan to use the whole batch immediately, feel free to skip this step.

Buffalo Shrimp Dip

Per Serving:

Calories	160
Fat	10g
Saturated Fat	6g
Cholesterol	110mg
Sodium	730mg
Carbohydrates	2g
Fiber	0g
Sugar	1g
Added Sugars	0g
Protein	14g

Enjoy a lightened up, low-carb version of a party classic for a delicious game day. Serve with lots of cut-up vegetables like cucumbers, peppers, carrots, celery, or cherry tomatoes.

4 ounces light cream cheese

¼ cup light sour cream

2 tablespoons buffalo hot sauce or sriracha

1 teaspoon white vinegar

½ cup shredded reduced-fat (2%) Mexican cheese, divided

1 (4-ounce) can baby shrimp, drained

1 Preheat oven to 350°F. Spray a small baking dish with nonstick cooking spray and set aside.
2 Soften cream cheese in a medium microwave-safe bowl about 20 seconds.
3 Add sour cream, hot sauce, and vinegar and stir well.
4 Add ¼ cup cheese and shrimp and gently stir to combine.
5 Transfer mixture to prepared baking dish and top with remaining ¼ cup cheese.
6 Bake 4–5 minutes. Turn on broiler and broil 2–3 minutes until cheese is melted, bubbly, and starting to brown.

Garlic Lovers Hummus

The ultimate vegetarian dip and sandwich spread. This version calls for tahini, a smooth sesame butter sold in many supermarkets and natural food stores. For a milder flavor, reduce the amount of garlic, and if you prefer, add ¼ teaspoon kosher salt.

1 (15-ounce) can low-sodium chickpeas, drained and rinsed

3 tablespoons sesame tahini

3 tablespoons lemon juice

2 tablespoons olive oil

4 medium cloves garlic, peeled

1 Place all ingredients into a food processor. Pulse until smooth.
2 Serve immediately or cover and refrigerate until serving.

MAKES 1½ CUPS	
Per Serving (2 tablespoons):	
Calories	70
Fat	5g
Saturated Fat	1g
Cholesterol	0mg
Sodium	40mg
Carbohydrates	5g
Fiber	2g
Sugar	1g
Added Sugars	0g
Protein	2g

Antipasto Salad

SERVES 8

Per Serving:

Calories	220
Fat	14g
Saturated Fat	4.5g
Cholesterol	20mg
Sodium	510mg
Carbohydrates	17g
Fiber	5g
Sugar	3g
Added Sugars	1g
Protein	10g

A perfect party starter, this hearty salad is packed with fiber-rich vegetables and beans. Feel free to switch up ingredients and cheeses to suit your pantry stock.

1 cup sliced (2" pieces) asparagus

1 cup thin strips yellow bell pepper

1 (14-ounce) can artichoke hearts, drained and quartered

1 (15.5-ounce) can low-sodium chickpeas, drained and rinsed

1 (14-ounce) can hearts of palm, drained and sliced into coins

¾ cup grape tomatoes

½ cup pitted kalamata olives

⅓ cup apple cider vinegar

2 tablespoons extra-virgin olive oil

1 tablespoon dried oregano

1 teaspoon sugar

¼ teaspoon kosher salt

¼ teaspoon ground black pepper

3 medium cloves garlic, peeled and minced

¼ cup chopped fresh parsley

8 ounces part-skim small mozzarella balls

1 Fill a medium saucepan halfway with water. Place over medium heat; bring to a boil. Next to saucepan, place a large bowl filled with water and ice. Add asparagus to boiling water. Blanch about 2 minutes, then remove from boiling water with a slotted spoon and place in ice water. Drain asparagus and pat dry with a towel.

2 In a large serving bowl, add asparagus, bell pepper, artichokes, chickpeas, hearts of palm, tomatoes, and olives.

3 In a small bowl, mix vinegar, oil, oregano, sugar, salt, black pepper, garlic, and parsley. Whisk well, pour over salad, and toss. Top with mozzarella and serve.

CHAPTER 4

Meat and Poultry

Soy and Ginger Flank Steak

The marinade in this dish is not only delicious, but it helps protect the meat from harmful compounds that are produced when grilling. Always marinate your meat for grilling when possible! This meat will need to marinate for at least 3–4 hours, so make sure to add that time into your planning.

SERVES 4	
Per Serving (4 ounces):	
Calories	210
Fat	8g
Saturated Fat	3g
Cholesterol	85mg
Sodium	80mg
Carbohydrates	0g
Fiber	0g
Sugar	0g
Added Sugars	0g
Protein	31g

1¼ pounds lean London broil

1 tablespoon minced fresh ginger

2 teaspoons minced garlic

1 tablespoon reduced-sodium soy sauce

3 tablespoons dry red wine

¼ teaspoon ground black pepper

½ tablespoon olive oil

1 Place steak, ginger, garlic, soy sauce, wine, black pepper, and oil in a medium shallow baking dish. Coat steak with marinade on both sides. Cover and refrigerate. Marinate at least 3–4 hours, turning once or twice so all marinade soaks into both sides of steak.

2 Heat a gas or charcoal grill. Place steak on grill and discard marinade. Grill steak, turning once during cooking, until done to your preference. Medium-rare will take approximately 12–15 minutes. Slice meat diagonally and against grain into thin slices. Serve.

SLICING MEATS AGAINST THE GRAIN

Certain cuts of meat such as flank steak, brisket, and London broil have a distinct grain (or line) of fibers running through them. If you slice with the grain, the meat will seem tough and difficult to chew. These cuts of meat should always be thinly sliced across (or against) the grain so the fibers are cut through and the meat remains tender and easy to chew.

Chipotle Chicken Wrap

Wraps are such an easy way to feed a family or a crowd when it's time for company. The high-fiber tortillas control the amount of carbs, and the heat from the chipotle and salsa can help burn a few extra calories too.

1 pound boneless, skinless chicken breast, cut into ½" strips

1 tablespoon lime juice

1 tablespoon olive oil

1 teaspoon chipotle seasoning

⅛ teaspoon ground black pepper

4 (8") high-fiber, low-carb flour tortillas

½ cup jarred salsa

1 cup chopped romaine lettuce

1 Place chicken, lime juice, oil, chipotle seasoning, and black pepper in a medium shallow dish. Turn to coat chicken fully in marinade. Cover and refrigerate 1 hour.

2 Heat a gas or charcoal grill.

3 Wrap tortillas in foil and place on grill's top rack. Place chicken on grill and cook 7–9 minutes until done, turning once during cooking.

4 Place chicken in center of each heated tortilla, add 2 tablespoons salsa to each, top with chopped lettuce, and wrap. Serve.

SERVES 4	
Per Serving:	
Calories	250
Fat	10g
Saturated Fat	2.5g
Cholesterol	85mg
Sodium	640mg
Carbohydrates	22g
Fiber	16g
Sugar	2g
Added Sugars	0g
Protein	31g

PUMP UP THE VEGETABLES

Wraps are so versatile and great vehicles to use up any extra vegetables in the refrigerator. You can top this chicken with roasted vegetables, avocado, jarred roasted peppers, or jalapeños. Use ramekins or muffin tins to display a variety of toppings for the family or guests to build their own wrap.

Tandoori-Style Chicken

GARAM MASALA

Garam masala is a combination of spices used in Indian cooking and can be found in many supermarkets. A basic recipe contains coriander, cinnamon, cloves, cardamom, and cumin. To make your own, try ½ teaspoon of each as a base and then make changes to suit your taste.

With only four ingredients, this simple dish brings the flavors of India to the dinner table. Serve with ½ cup brown basmati rice and your favorite vegetables.

1½ pounds boneless, skinless chicken breast halves, pounded thin

1 tablespoon garam masala

2 large cloves garlic, peeled and finely chopped

½ cup plain nonfat Greek yogurt

1 Place chicken, garam masala, garlic, and yogurt in a medium shallow dish. Turn to coat chicken fully in marinade. Cover and refrigerate at least 3–4 hours or overnight.

2 Preheat broiler. Place chicken on a medium baking sheet lightly coated with nonstick cooking spray.

3 Broil chicken on top rack 4–5 minutes per side until internal temperature reaches 165°F. Serve.

Chicken Lo Mein

Chinese takeout is typically very high in sodium and contains a lot of oil. This homemade version of Chicken Lo Mein brings all the flavors with a much improved nutrition profile.

2½ tablespoons reduced-sodium soy sauce, divided

1 teaspoon grated fresh ginger

1 tablespoon unflavored rice vinegar

¼ teaspoon ground turmeric

1 pound boneless, skinless chicken breast, cut into 1" cubes

½ tablespoon canola oil

½ cup sliced scallions

2 teaspoons minced garlic

3 cups shredded coleslaw mix

¼ teaspoon red pepper flakes

2 cups cooked whole-grain spaghetti

1 teaspoon sesame oil

1 teaspoon sesame seeds

SERVES 4	
Per Serving:	
Calories	310
Fat	8g
Saturated Fat	1g
Cholesterol	85mg
Sodium	430mg
Carbohydrates	27g
Fiber	4g
Sugar	2g
Added Sugars	0g
Protein	31g

1 In a medium bowl, combine 1½ tablespoons soy sauce, ginger, rice vinegar, and turmeric. Mix in cubed chicken and set aside.
2 Heat canola oil in a large skillet or wok over medium heat and sauté scallions and garlic 1 minute. Add chicken and cook quickly until meat and scallions are slightly browned, about 8–10 minutes.
3 Add coleslaw to skillet and continue to stir-fry another 3–4 minutes. Sprinkle in red pepper flakes.
4 When vegetables are crisp-tender, add cooked pasta, sesame oil, remaining 1 tablespoon soy sauce, and sesame seeds. Toss lightly and serve.

Chicken Piccata

An Italian staple made easy at home. The sauce in this dish is so delicious you might find yourself licking it up! Serve with sautéed spinach or broccoli and a serving of a whole grain or roasted potatoes.

1 tablespoon olive oil

1 teaspoon unsalted butter

4 (4-ounce) boneless, skinless chicken breasts

½ teaspoon kosher salt

¼ teaspoon ground black pepper

1½ tablespoons white whole-wheat flour

⅔ cup low-sodium chicken broth

¼ cup dry white wine

3 tablespoons lemon juice

¼ cup chopped fresh parsley

1 tablespoon jarred capers, drained

1 In a large skillet over medium-high heat, heat oil and butter.
2 Sprinkle tops of chicken evenly with salt, black pepper, and flour. Add chicken, flour side down, to skillet and cook 4 minutes on each side or until cooked through.
3 Remove chicken from skillet and set aside. Add broth, wine, and lemon juice to skillet, reduce heat, and simmer 2–3 minutes until sauce thickens slightly.
4 Stir in parsley and capers. Place chicken back in skillet approximately 2 minutes to heat through. Serve.

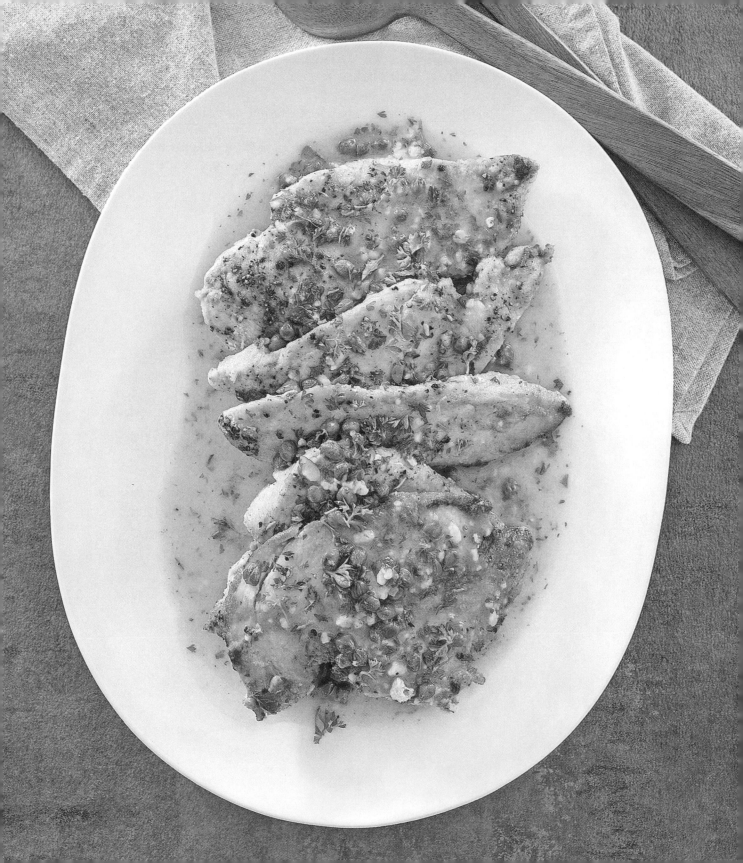

Chicken Cacciatore

Per Serving:

Calories	260
Fat	6g
Saturated Fat	1g
Cholesterol	85mg
Sodium	100mg
Carbohydrates	17g
Fiber	2g
Sugar	8g
Added Sugars	2g
Protein	30g

The beauty of this tried-and-true family favorite is the ease of preparation. For a gluten-free recipe, simply leave out the flour or use a gluten-free variety to dredge the chicken. Enjoy this over ½ cup of any whole grain such as whole-wheat pasta, freekeh, farro, brown or black rice, quinoa, or sorghum.

¼ cup white whole-wheat flour

⅛ teaspoon ground black pepper

1½ pounds boneless, skinless thin chicken breasts, cut into 4-ounce pieces

2 teaspoons extra-virgin olive oil

2 small green bell peppers, seeded and sliced into ¼" strips

12 ounces white mushrooms, sliced

1 (25-ounce) jar low-sodium marinara sauce

½ cup dry red wine

1 Place flour and black pepper in a medium shallow bowl. Dredge chicken on both sides in flour and then discard extra.

2 Heat a large saucepan with lid over medium-high heat and add oil. Add chicken and sauté 3 minutes per side.

3 On top of chicken, add green peppers, mushrooms, marinara sauce, and wine. Cover, reduce heat, and simmer 20 minutes or until vegetables are cooked and sauce is reduced. Serve.

Easy Turkey Bolognese

This simple dinner comes together in the time it takes to boil water and cook pasta. Adding ground mushrooms extends the dish and provides extra nutrition even for the pickiest of eaters. Serve this dish over whole-wheat pasta, bean-based pasta, or zoodles.

8 ounces white mushrooms, quartered

1⅓ pounds 93% lean ground turkey

1 (25-ounce) jar low-sodium marinara sauce

¼ teaspoon ground black pepper

¼ teaspoon garlic powder

¼ teaspoon dried oregano

½ teaspoon kosher salt

¼ cup grated Parmesan cheese

1 Place mushrooms into a food processor or blender. Pulse until ground.

2 Spray a large pot with nonstick cooking spray over medium-high heat. Add turkey and ground mushrooms side by side. Do not disturb for 5 minutes, then break up turkey and combine with mushrooms, stirring until cooked through, about 3–5 more minutes.

3 Stir in marinara sauce and seasonings, reduce heat to low, and cook an additional 5–10 minutes to reduce. Sprinkle with Parmesan and serve.

SERVES 6

Per Serving:	
Calories	220
Fat	12g
Saturated Fat	2.5g
Cholesterol	50mg
Sodium	340mg
Carbohydrates	9g
Fiber	2g
Sugar	5g
Added Sugars	0g
Protein	26g

MUSHROOMS AS A MEAT EXTENDER

Mushrooms are unique as they take on the flavor, color, and texture of ground beef or turkey when blended and added to a dish. This allows for extra vegetables and less meat per serving, adding to the nutritional value and saving money as well.

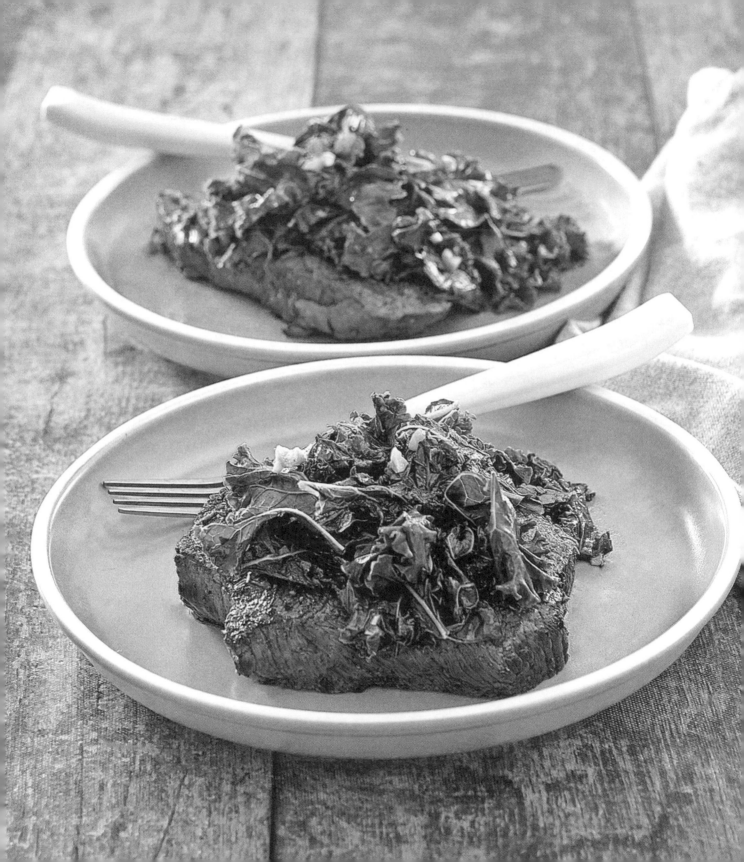

Seared Sirloin Steaks with Garlicky Greens

This juicy, medium-rare beef accented with tart and tangy kale is certain to impress guests. If you prefer you could also use Swiss chard. Serve with roasted potatoes or your favorite whole grain for a spectacular meal in a snap.

1½ pounds sirloin steak (1" thick), trimmed and cut into 6 pieces

1 tablespoon coarsely chopped fresh rosemary

½ teaspoon ground black pepper, divided

1 tablespoon olive oil

¾ cup dry white wine

4 medium cloves garlic, peeled and minced

2 tablespoons white balsamic vinegar

1 teaspoon sugar

1 teaspoon Dijon mustard

1½ pounds kale, trimmed and coarsely chopped, stems discarded

SERVES 6	
Per Serving:	
Calories	330
Fat	13g
Saturated Fat	4g
Cholesterol	100mg
Sodium	450mg
Carbohydrates	13g
Fiber	4g
Sugar	5g
Added Sugars	1g
Protein	39g

1 Preheat oven to 400°F. Line a medium rimmed baking sheet with aluminum foil and set aside.

2 Season both sides of steaks with rosemary and ¼ teaspoon black pepper.

3 In a medium skillet over medium-high heat, heat oil. Place steaks in skillet and cook until nicely browned, 3–4 minutes per side.

4 Remove from heat and transfer steaks to prepared baking sheet. Place on middle rack in oven and roast 5 minutes. Remove from oven and set aside.

5 Return skillet to medium-high heat. Add wine and cook, scraping up browned bits from bottom of skillet, 3 minutes. Add garlic, vinegar, sugar, mustard, and remaining ¼ teaspoon black pepper and stir to combine.

6 Add kale and toss well to coat. Cover skillet and cook, stirring once or twice, until tender, about 5 minutes.

7 Transfer steaks to six medium plates and top with kale. Serve immediately.

Turkey Meatloaf Muffins

A fun twist on meatloaf, these "muffins" will get two thumbs up from the whole family. The smaller potions cook quicker than a full meatloaf and allow for easy serving. Try "icing" your meatloaf muffins with Mashed Cauliflower (see Chapter 6).

1 pound 93% lean ground turkey

1 large egg

⅓ cup Homemade High-Fiber Bread Crumbs (see Chapter 9)

¼ teaspoon garlic powder

¼ teaspoon ground black pepper

3 tablespoons no-sugar-added ketchup

1½ teaspoons Worcestershire sauce

2 ounces white mushrooms, diced small (about 2 large)

2 tablespoons low-fat milk

3 tablespoons dehydrated onions

½ teaspoon Dijon mustard

1 Preheat oven to 350°F. Spray a twelve-cup muffin tin with non-stick cooking spray or line with liners.

2 In a large bowl, combine all ingredients. Divide mixture into prepared muffin cups (about ¼ cup each).

3 Bake approximately 30 minutes or until internal temperature reaches 165°F. Serve.

Southwest Black Bean Burgers

Beans are not only a great meat extender to save you money but they also add fiber and plant-based protein to your burgers. Enjoy these patties as traditional burgers or crumble one up on a taco salad with lots of vegetables and avocado for even more fiber and heart-healthy fat.

1 cup canned low-sodium black beans, drained and rinsed

¼ cup chopped red onion

1 teaspoon chili powder

1 teaspoon ground cumin

2 tablespoons minced fresh parsley

¼ teaspoon kosher salt

1 pound lean ground beef

SERVES 5	
Per Serving:	
Calories	210
Fat	9g
Saturated Fat	3.5g
Cholesterol	60mg
Sodium	200mg
Carbohydrates	9g
Fiber	4g
Sugar	1g
Added Sugars	0g
Protein	21g

1 In a food processor, place beans, onion, chili powder, cumin, parsley, and salt. Combine ingredients using pulse setting until beans are partially puréed and all ingredients are mixed.

2 In a medium bowl, combine ground beef and bean mixture. Shape into five patties.

3 Meat mixture will be quite soft after mixing, so place patties on a tray and freeze for a few minutes prior to cooking.

4 Heat a medium stovetop grill pan or gas or charcoal grill to high heat, and brush with oil to prevent sticking. Grill burgers approximately 6 minutes on each side, until internal temperature reaches 160°F. Serve.

London Broil with Grilled Vegetables

SERVES 2	
Per Serving:	
Calories	370
Fat	10g
Saturated Fat	3.5g
Cholesterol	85mg
Sodium	115mg
Carbohydrates	35g
Fiber	6g
Sugar	23g
Added Sugars	0g
Protein	37g

Steak and vegetables are made simple and delicious in this meal. Serve with a big salad and ½ cup brown rice or your favorite whole grain. If using wooden skewers, soak them for 30 minutes to avoid burning them.

2 tablespoons olive oil

1 teaspoon red wine vinegar

1 tablespoon steak sauce

½ teaspoon red pepper flakes

1 medium zucchini, cut into 1" chunks

1 medium orange or yellow bell pepper, seeded and cut into quarters

2 medium sweet onions, peeled and cut into thick chunks

4 cherry tomatoes

8 ounces London broil, cut into chunks

1 In a medium bowl, mix oil, vinegar, steak sauce, and red pepper flakes.
2 Place zucchini, bell pepper, onions, and tomatoes on a medium plate and brush with dressing.
3 Add meat to bowl and toss with remaining dressing to coat.
4 Using four metal barbecue skewers, skewer vegetables and London broil, alternating between meat and different vegetables.
5 Heat a gas or charcoal grill to high and grill vegetables and meat, turning every few minutes to desired level of doneness, about 12–15 minutes.

Chicken Breasts in Balsamic Vinegar Sauce

Balsamic vinegar is so powerful it allows for less oil and sodium in this flavorful dish. Serve with Mashed Cauliflower (see Chapter 6) and a vegetable like broccoli, mushrooms, or asparagus.

4 (5-ounce) boneless, skinless chicken breasts, pounded even

¼ teaspoon kosher salt

⅛ teaspoon ground black pepper

1 tablespoon whipped butter

1 tablespoon olive oil

¼ cup chopped red onion

2 teaspoons finely chopped garlic

3 tablespoons balsamic vinegar

1½ cups low-sodium chicken broth

½ teaspoon dried oregano

SERVES 4	
Per Serving:	
Calories	240
Fat	9g
Saturated Fat	2.5g
Cholesterol	105mg
Sodium	180mg
Carbohydrates	4g
Fiber	0g
Sugar	2g
Added Sugars	0g
Protein	33g

1 Sprinkle chicken on both sides with salt and black pepper.

2 Heat butter and oil in a large skillet over medium heat. Add chicken and cook until browned, about 5 minutes per side. Reduce heat and cook a few more minutes until chicken is cooked through. Transfer to a medium platter, cover, and keep warm.

3 To the skillet, add onion and garlic and sauté over medium heat 3 minutes, scraping up browned bits.

4 Add vinegar and bring to a boil. Boil up to 3 minutes or until reduced to a glaze, stirring constantly.

5 Add broth and boil until liquid is reduced by about half. Stir in oregano. Return chicken to skillet to heat through, about 1–2 minutes. Spoon sauce over chicken and serve immediately.

Ginger and Garlic Pork Stir-Fry

Intensely flavorful and speedy to prepare, this stir-fry features tender pork loin and crisp vegetables in a delectable sauce. Serve over cooked brown rice or whole-wheat angel hair pasta.

SERVES 4

Per Serving:

Calories	170
Fat	4g
Saturated Fat	1g
Cholesterol	35mg
Sodium	440mg
Carbohydrates	17g
Fiber	5g
Sugar	7g
Added Sugars	0g
Protein	17g

QUICK COOK TIP

Cut your prep time by using a bag of frozen stir-fry vegetables in place of the snap peas, carrots, peppers, and onions.

8 ounces pork tenderloin, thinly sliced

1½ tablespoons minced fresh ginger

3 medium cloves garlic, peeled and minced

2 tablespoons light soy sauce

¾ cup low-sodium vegetable broth

2 teaspoons cornstarch

2 teaspoons sesame oil

1 medium head bok choy, sliced

8 ounces pea pods or sugar snap peas

2 medium carrots, peeled and sliced

1 medium red bell pepper, seeded and diced

1 small red onion, peeled and diced

4 medium scallions, sliced

¼ teaspoon ground black pepper

1 In a large bowl, add pork, ginger, garlic, and soy sauce and stir well to coat. Set aside.
2 In a medium bowl, add broth and cornstarch and whisk well to combine. Set aside.
3 Heat oil in a large frying pan or wok over medium heat 1 minute. Add bok choy, pea pods, carrots, bell pepper, and red onion and cook, stirring, 5 minutes.
4 Add pork mixture and cook, stirring, 3 minutes.
5 Add broth mixture and cook, stirring, until sauce thickens, approximately 30 seconds to 1 minute.
6 Remove from heat. Stir in scallions and season with black pepper. Serve immediately.

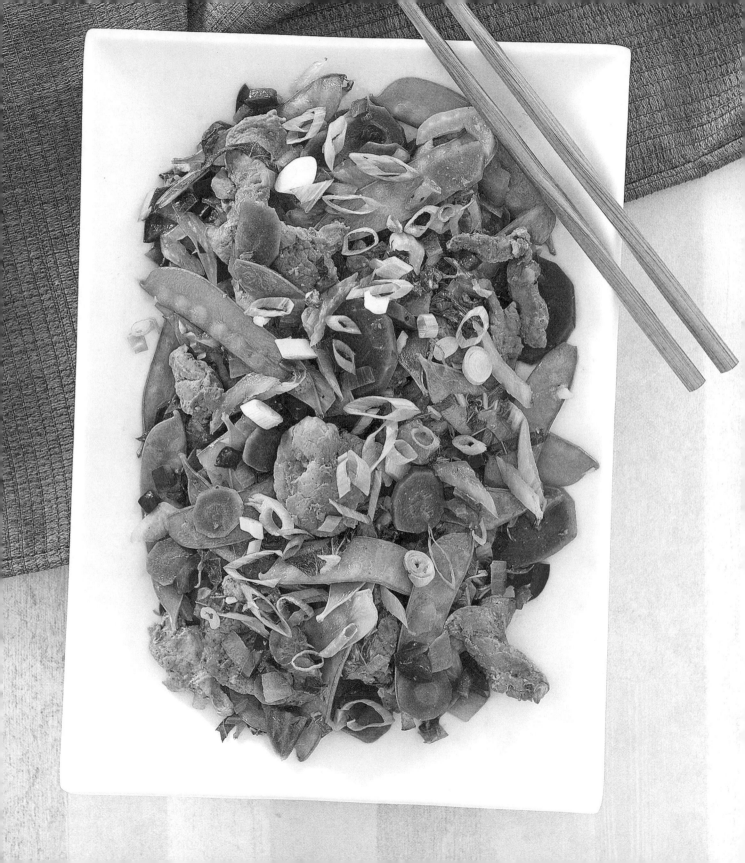

One-Pot Herbed Chicken and Brown Rice

SERVES 4

Per Serving:

Calories	390
Fat	9g
Saturated Fat	1.5g
Cholesterol	105mg
Sodium	125mg
Carbohydrates	40g
Fiber	2g
Sugar	0g
Added Sugars	0g
Protein	37g

Chicken and rice is about as simple as it gets, and using instant brown rice sharply cuts down on the cooking time. Only a few pantry ingredients are needed to whip up this one-pot dinner, or you can toss in a steamer bag of vegetables for extra nutrients and fiber.

1 tablespoon olive oil

4 (5-ounce) boneless, skinless chicken breasts

⅛ teaspoon kosher salt

⅛ teaspoon ground black pepper

¾ teaspoon garlic powder, divided

¾ teaspoon dried rosemary, divided

1½ cups low-sodium chicken broth

2 cups uncooked instant brown rice

1 In a large nonstick skillet over medium-high heat, heat oil.

2 Sprinkle one side of chicken with salt and black pepper. Add chicken to skillet, salt and pepper side down, and sprinkle with half of garlic powder and half of rosemary. Cover and cook 4 minutes on each side or until cooked through. Remove chicken from skillet and set aside.

3 Add broth to skillet and stir to deglaze pan and bring to a boil. Stir in rice and remaining garlic powder and rosemary. Top with chicken and cover. Reduce heat to low and cook 5 minutes. Remove from heat and let stand, covered, 5 minutes before serving.

Hoisin Chicken Lettuce Wraps

This DIY restaurant favorite is a fun and flavorful lower-carb appetizer or entrée. Add some riced cauliflower to pack in even more vegetables.

1 tablespoon olive oil

1 pound lean ground chicken

2 large cloves garlic, peeled and minced

1 medium onion, peeled and diced

¼ cup hoisin sauce

2 tablespoons light soy sauce

1 tablespoon unflavored rice wine vinegar

1 (1") piece fresh ginger, grated

½ teaspoon sriracha

1 (8-ounce) can water chestnuts, drained and diced

3 medium scallions, thinly sliced, divided

8 large lettuce leaves (like butter, Bibb, or Boston)

1 In a medium saucepan over medium-high heat, heat oil.

2 Add chicken and cook until browned, 3–5 minutes, crumbling it as it cooks.

3 Stir in garlic, onion, hoisin sauce, soy sauce, vinegar, ginger, and sriracha. Cook 1–2 minutes until onion becomes translucent.

4 Stir in water chestnuts and two-thirds of scallions and cook until tender, 1–2 minutes.

5 Spoon a few tablespoons of chicken mixture into center of each lettuce leaf and sprinkle with remaining scallions to serve.

SERVES 4

Per Serving (2 lettuce wraps):

Calories	290
Fat	15g
Saturated Fat	.5g
Cholesterol	55mg
Sodium	670mg
Carbohydrates	15g
Fiber	2g
Sugar	7g
Added Sugars	0g
Protein	22g

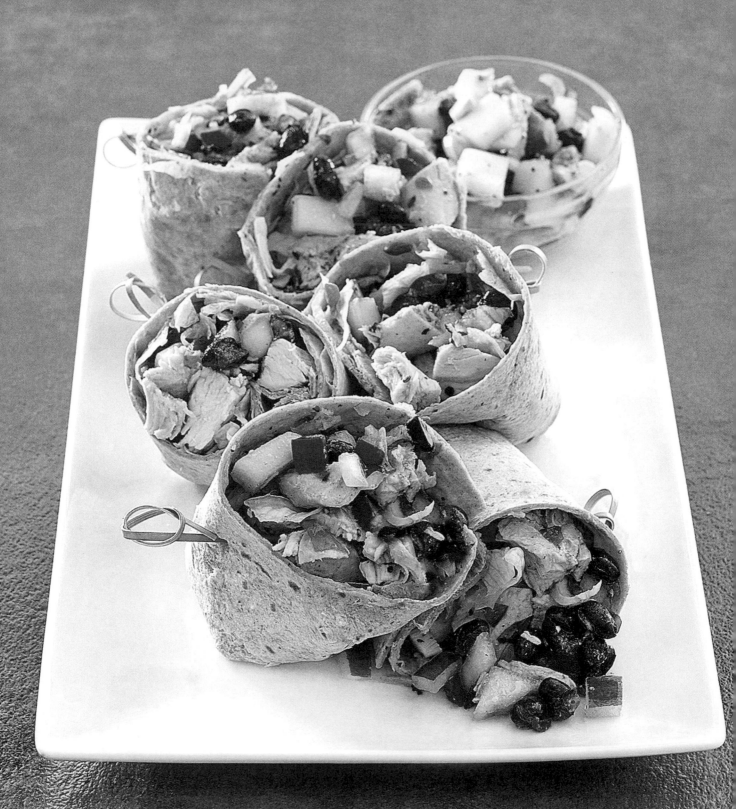

Tropical Chicken Salad Wrap Sandwiches

Colorfully festive with a fresh, spicy kick, these sandwiches make great party fare. This filling swaps out the traditional mayonnaise in favor of a light vinaigrette. Look for a high-fiber flatbread that contains 90–110 calories. For even more flavor and color, try this on a spinach or tomato-basil wrap.

1 pound rotisserie chicken, cut into bite-sized cubes

1 medium ripe mango, peeled, pitted, and diced

1 small red onion, peeled and diced

1 small bell pepper, seeded and diced

1 medium jalapeño pepper, seeded and minced

2 medium cloves garlic, peeled and minced

1 cup canned low-sodium black beans, drained and rinsed

2 tablespoons apple cider vinegar

Juice of 1 medium lime (about 2 tablespoons)

2 tablespoons olive oil

¼ cup chopped fresh cilantro

½ teaspoon ground black pepper

4 cups mixed salad greens

6 high-fiber flatbreads or 8" high-fiber, low-carb flour tortillas

1 In a large bowl, add chicken, mango, onion, bell pepper, jalapeño, garlic, and beans and mix.

2 In a small bowl, add vinegar, lime juice, oil, cilantro, and black pepper and whisk well to combine. Pour over chicken salad and stir well to coat.

3 Divide greens and chicken salad evenly between flatbreads, then roll sandwiches up. Slice each in half using a sharp knife.

4 Serve immediately or cover and refrigerate until ready to serve.

SERVES 6	
Per Serving:	
Calories	300
Fat	10g
Saturated Fat	2.5g
Cholesterol	65mg
Sodium	650mg
Carbohydrates	37g
Fiber	19g
Sugar	7g
Added Sugars	2g
Protein	30g

Grilled Lamb Chops with Garlic, Rosemary, and Thyme

SERVES 2

Per Serving:

Calories	250
Fat	15g
Saturated Fat	4g
Cholesterol	85mg
Sodium	370mg
Carbohydrates	1g
Fiber	0g
Sugar	0g
Added Sugars	0g
Protein	27g

Lamb chops feel fancy yet are very easy to prepare. The herb and spice combo used here is refreshingly tasty.

2 medium cloves garlic, peeled
½ teaspoon kosher salt
1 teaspoon chopped fresh rosemary
1 teaspoon chopped fresh thyme
1 tablespoon olive oil
1 teaspoon lemon zest
1/16 teaspoon ground black pepper
4 (1¼"-thick) lamb chops

1 In a medium bowl, mash garlic cloves into a paste. Add salt and stir.
2 Add rosemary, thyme, oil, lemon zest, and black pepper and stir well to combine.
3 Rub herb and garlic paste onto lamb and set aside to marinate 10 minutes.
4 Heat a gas or charcoal grill to high heat. Place lamb on grill and grill 4–5 minutes on each side for medium-rare doneness. Serve.

Pesto Spaghetti Squash with Chicken, Tomatoes, and Feta

Whip up this hearty, flavorful, and satisfying low-carb meal in a flash with just a few simple ingredients.

2 tablespoons Walnut Pesto Sauce (see Chapter 3)

1 cup cooked spaghetti squash, warm

3 ounces rotisserie chicken breast, cut into bite-sized pieces

½ cup halved cherry or grape tomatoes

2 tablespoons crumbled feta cheese

⅛ teaspoon ground black pepper

1 In a medium serving bowl, stir Pesto Sauce into warmed spaghetti squash until evenly distributed.

2 Add chicken, tomatoes, and feta and toss to combine. Season with black pepper and serve.

SERVES 1	
Per Serving:	
Calories	390
Fat	24g
Saturated Fat	6g
Cholesterol	95mg
Sodium	790mg
Carbohydrates	20g
Fiber	3g
Sugar	6g
Added Sugars	0g
Protein	31g

Oven-Baked Chicken Tenders

SERVES 4

Per Serving:

Calories	280
Fat	5g
Saturated Fat	1g
Cholesterol	125mg
Sodium	120mg
Carbohydrates	16g
Fiber	4g
Sugar	1g
Added Sugars	0g
Protein	42g

Baked rather than fried, these crispy tenders are much lower in fat, but have a whole lot of flavor. These also freeze wonderfully—just place leftovers into an airtight container for later meals.

½ cup white whole-wheat flour

¼ cup Homemade High-Fiber Bread Crumbs (see Chapter 9)

1 teaspoon garlic powder

1 teaspoon onion powder

½ teaspoon ground sweet paprika

½ teaspoon ground black pepper

¼ cup 1% milk

1 large egg white

1½ pounds boneless, skinless chicken breast tenderloins

1 Preheat oven to 375°F. Line a large baking sheet with nonstick aluminum foil, spray lightly with nonstick cooking spray, and set aside.

2 In a large zip-top plastic bag, combine flour, Homemade High-Fiber Bread Crumbs, garlic powder, onion powder, paprika, and black pepper. Seal and shake well to combine.

3 In a small shallow bowl, whisk milk and egg white.

4 One piece at a time, dip chicken into milk mixture, then place in flour bag, seal, and shake to coat. Place breaded tenders on prepared baking sheet and spray tops with nonstick cooking spray.

5 Place baking sheet on middle rack in oven and bake 10–15 minutes until golden brown and cooked through. Remove from oven and serve immediately.

CHAPTER 5

Fish and Seafood

Garlic Shrimp with Bok Choy

Per Serving:

Calories	190
Fat	6g
Saturated Fat	1g
Cholesterol	210mg
Sodium	650mg
Carbohydrates	7g
Fiber	2g
Sugar	2g
Added Sugars	0g
Protein	31g

BOK CHOY

Bok choy is a Chinese cabbage that is staggeringly simple to prepare and is rich in many important nutrients including vitamin A, vitamin C, and folate. Serve over ½ cup of brown rice or riced cauliflower to add even more vegetables to your meal.

Frozen shrimp are one of the handiest freezer staples. Defrost them under running water for a few minutes and they cook just as quickly as fresh shrimp. This dish comes together fast for busy weeknights—serve it with riced cauliflower for a low-carb option or with ½ cup of brown rice per person for extra fiber.

1 tablespoon sesame oil

3 large cloves garlic, peeled and chopped

2 teaspoons grated fresh ginger

1 pound bok choy, chopped

1 cup broccoli florets

1 pound shrimp, shelled and deveined

2 tablespoons reduced-sodium soy sauce

1 teaspoon sesame seeds

1. Heat oil in a medium skillet or wok over medium-high heat. Add garlic and ginger, stir, and cook 30 seconds.
2. Turn heat to high. Add bok choy and broccoli and stir-fry 2–3 minutes. Add shrimp and continue stirring.
3. Add soy sauce and cook until shrimp are pink and completely done. Garnish with sesame seeds and serve.

Shrimp Tacos with Creamy Slaw

This healthier version of soft tacos is made much lower in fat and carbs by swapping Greek yogurt for sour cream and using a high-fiber tortilla. If you can, grill the shrimp on skewers for extra deliciousness.

¼ cup light mayonnaise

½ cup plain nonfat Greek yogurt

¼ cup chopped onion

2 tablespoons minced jalapeño pepper

2 teaspoons minced fresh cilantro

⅛ teaspoon kosher salt

2 cups shredded green cabbage

¼ cup lime juice

1 medium clove garlic, peeled and minced

1 tablespoon canola oil

1 pound large shrimp, shelled and deveined

4 (8") high-fiber, low-carb flour tortillas

1 cup chopped tomato

⅛ teaspoon ground black pepper

SERVES 4	
Per Serving:	
Calories	280
Fat	11g
Saturated Fat	2g
Cholesterol	190mg
Sodium	630mg
Carbohydrates	28g
Fiber	17g
Sugar	4g
Added Sugars	0g
Protein	32g

1 In a medium bowl, whisk together mayonnaise, yogurt, onion, jalapeño, cilantro, and salt. Stir in cabbage and place in refrigerator to chill.

2 In a large bowl, combine lime juice, garlic, and oil to make a marinade for shrimp. Add shrimp to bowl and stir to combine. Cover and refrigerate at least 1 hour.

3 Heat a medium sauté pan over medium-high heat and spray with nonstick cooking spray. With a slotted spoon, remove shrimp from marinade, add to pan, and sauté until cooked through, about 3–5 minutes. Discard marinade.

4 While shrimp is cooking, warm tortillas on a medium plate about 20 seconds in microwave.

5 To assemble tacos, divide shrimp into four portions. Place a portion in center of each heated tortilla. Top with cabbage mixture and tomatoes. Add black pepper and serve.

Mediterranean Salmon Salad with Artichokes, White Beans, and Lemon Dressing

Per Serving:

Calories	200
Fat	5g
Saturated Fat	0.5g
Cholesterol	40mg
Sodium	614mg
Carbohydrates	16g
Fiber	4g
Sugar	3g
Added Sugars	0g
Protein	23g

Meet your seafood goals without turning on the oven. This low-carb, gluten-free salad makes a fabulous light lunch or dinner. Swap in tuna for salmon if you prefer.

2 (6-ounce) cans skinless, boneless salmon

½ small red onion, peeled and diced

½ cup canned low-sodium small white beans, drained and rinsed

1 (14-ounce) can artichokes, rinsed, patted dry, and separated into leaves

2 tablespoons chopped fresh parsley, plus more for garnish

1 large clove garlic, peeled and finely chopped

1 tablespoon extra-virgin olive oil

¼ cup lemon juice

1 teaspoon lemon zest

½ teaspoon kosher salt

½ teaspoon ground black pepper

1 In a medium bowl, add salmon, onion, beans, artichokes, and parsley and gently combine.

2 In a small bowl add garlic, oil, lemon juice, lemon zest, salt, and black pepper and whisk to blend.

3 Pour dressing over salmon mixture and gently stir to make sure it's evenly distributed. For best flavor, cover and refrigerate at least 30 minutes before serving.

A-Taste-of-Italy Baked Fish

White mild fish like cod is enhanced beautifully by Italian flavors and spices. This basic dish can be served over whole-grain or bean-based pasta for a fiber boost or with sautéed spinach for a lower-carb meal.

1 (14.5-ounce) can stewed tomatoes, undrained

¼ teaspoon dried minced onion

½ teaspoon dried minced garlic

¼ teaspoon dried basil

¼ teaspoon dried parsley

⅛ teaspoon dried oregano

⅛ teaspoon sugar

1 tablespoon grated Parmesan cheese

1½ pounds cod fillets, patted dry

1 Preheat oven to 375°F.
2 In a medium baking pan or casserole dish coated with nonstick cooking spray, combine all ingredients except fillets and mix together.
3 Arrange fillets over mixture, folding thin tail ends under. Spoon some of the mixture over fillets. For fillets about 1" thick, bake uncovered 20–25 minutes or until fish is opaque and flaky. Serve.

SERVES 4	
Per Serving:	
Calories	170
Fat	2g
Saturated Fat	0.5g
Cholesterol	75mg
Sodium	330mg
Carbohydrates	6g
Fiber	1g
Sugar	5g
Added Sugars	2g
Protein	32g

Mussels Fra Diavolo

SERVES 4

Per Serving:

Calories	330
Fat	8g
Saturated Fat	1g
Cholesterol	20mg
Sodium	380mg
Carbohydrates	51g
Fiber	8g
Sugar	8g
Added Sugars	0g
Protein	16g

FRA DIAVOLO

If it's difficult to find fra diavolo sauce, use marinara and add red pepper flakes to suit your heat preference. There are several brands of low-sodium fra diavolo or arrabbiata sauce on the market, which will still taste delicious and will significantly lower the sodium per serving, so be sure to check the nutrition labels.

Serve an affordable, hearty, home-cooked seafood dinner in a flash with this tasty, four-ingredient dish. If you don't love angel hair pasta, feel free to substitute any fiber-rich pasta of your choice.

2 pounds fresh mussels (preferably Prince Edward Island)

8 ounces dry whole-wheat angel hair pasta

1 (25-ounce) jar low-sodium fra diavolo pasta sauce

¼ cup chopped fresh basil

1　In a large colander, thoroughly rinse and inspect mussels, discarding any cracked or open shells and making sure to debeard any mussels still holding on to one.

2　Start to cook pasta according to instructions on the box.

3　While pasta is cooking, place mussels in a large pot with lid. Cover and turn heat to high, checking occasionally until mussels open, approximately 3–5 minutes.

4　Remove mussels from heat, drain any extra liquid out of pot, and discard any unopened shells.

5　Return pot to stove over low to medium heat, add fra diavolo sauce to mussels, and heat through 2–3 minutes.

6　To serve add approximately 1 cup cooked pasta to bowls and distribute mussels and sauce on top. Garnish with fresh basil.

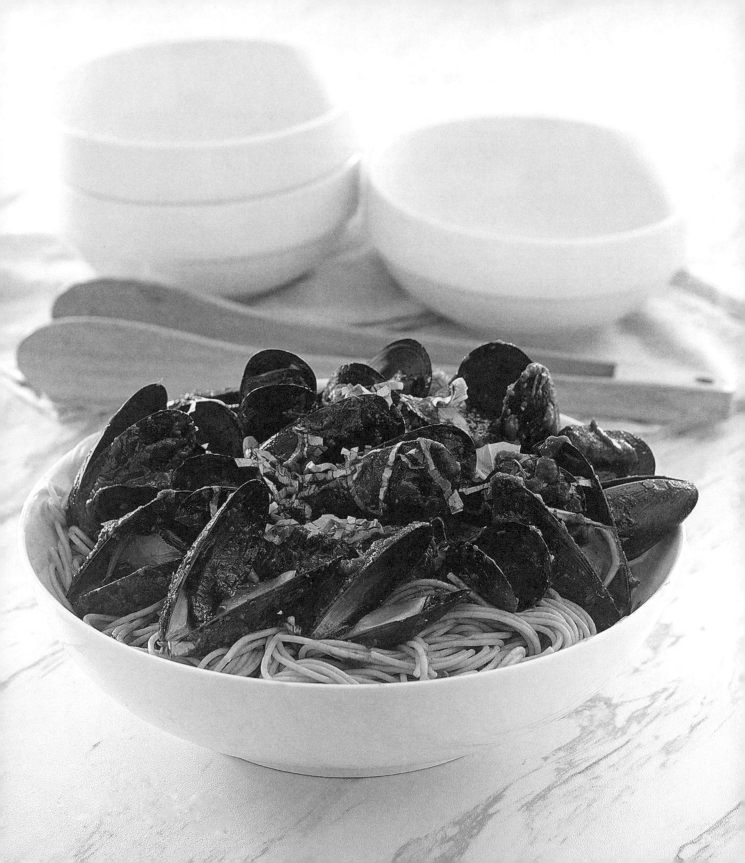

Baked Tuna Cakes

SERVES 4	
Per Serving:	
Calories	160
Fat	7g
Saturated Fat	1.5g
Cholesterol	80mg
Sodium	250mg
Carbohydrates	8g
Fiber	3g
Sugar	2g
Added Sugars	0g
Protein	17g

If you love crab cakes, try these tuna cakes for an easy and less expensive way to get your recommended two servings of fish per week. Serve over a salad, in a high-fiber wrap with tzatziki, lettuce, and tomato, or over a bed of roasted vegetables.

2 (5-ounce) cans water-packed no-salt-added solid white tuna, drained

1 small carrot, peeled and shredded

1 small stalk celery, finely diced

1 medium shallot, peeled and finely chopped

2 medium cloves garlic, peeled and minced

1 large egg

½ cup Homemade High-Fiber Bread Crumbs (see Chapter 9)

2 tablespoons light mayonnaise

½ teaspoon dried dill

½ teaspoon dried thyme

¼ teaspoon ground rosemary

⅛ teaspoon ground black pepper

1 Preheat oven to 400°F. Spray a medium baking sheet with non-stick cooking spray and set aside.

2 Drain tuna and place in a medium mixing bowl. Add remaining ingredients and stir well to combine.

3 Shape mixture into four equal patties and place on prepared baking sheet.

4 Place baking sheet on middle rack in oven and bake 10 minutes. Remove from oven, gently flip, and bake 5 minutes more. Remove from oven and serve immediately.

Pistachio-Crusted Salmon

While bread crumbs can be soggy when you try to coat moist fish, pistachios are guaranteed to give you fabulous flavor and a satisfying crunch. This nutty recipe pairs well with a side of sweet potatoes and veggies.

1 cup shelled pistachios

1 teaspoon chopped garlic

2 tablespoons chopped fresh basil

1 teaspoon dried thyme

1 teaspoon dried rosemary

¼ teaspoon kosher salt

¼ teaspoon ground black pepper

6 (4-ounce) salmon fillets

1 tablespoon honey

1. Preheat oven to 375°F. Spray a medium baking pan with nonstick cooking spray and set aside.

2. In a small food processor, grind pistachios, garlic, basil, thyme, rosemary, salt, and black pepper. Transfer mixture to a medium plate.

3. Brush top of each fillet with ½ teaspoon honey. Press honey-coated side into pistachio mixture.

4. Place salmon pistachio side up on prepared pan. Bake 15–17 minutes until fillets flake with a fork. Serve.

Cajun Catfish

SERVES 4

Per Serving:

Calories	140
Fat	7g
Saturated Fat	1.5g
Cholesterol	60mg
Sodium	180mg
Carbohydrates	1g
Fiber	1g
Sugar	0g
Added Sugars	0g
Protein	18g

A hint of New Orleans in your kitchen, this fish is fairly foolproof. Adjust the spice level up or down to suit your heat tolerance.

2 teaspoons ground paprika

1 teaspoon dried oregano

¼ teaspoon kosher salt

¼ teaspoon garlic powder

¼ teaspoon ground black pepper

¼ teaspoon ground cayenne pepper

1 pound catfish fillets

1 tablespoon lemon juice

1 Place a medium skillet sprayed with nonstick cooking spray over medium-high heat.

2 In a small bowl, combine paprika, oregano, salt, garlic powder, black pepper, and cayenne and mix well.

3 Brush both sides of fish with lemon juice and sprinkle ½ teaspoon of seasoning on each side.

4 Place fish in hot skillet, cover, and sauté 3–5 minutes on each side until fish flakes easily with a fork. Serve.

Roasted Salmon with Lemon, Mustard, and Dill

Salmon is best without a lot of fanfare. Here it's roasted simply with a delectably tart and tangy dill glaze.

1¼ pounds salmon, cut into 4 fillets

3 tablespoons lemon juice (from 1 large lemon)

2 tablespoons brown or Dijon mustard

2 tablespoons chopped fresh dill

⅛ teaspoon ground black pepper

1 Preheat oven to 450°F. Spray a medium baking pan with nonstick cooking spray.

2 Arrange fillets in baking pan.

3 In a small bowl, combine remaining ingredients and brush tops and sides of fillets with mixture. Drizzle any remaining mixture over fillets.

4 Place pan on middle rack in oven and bake 10–15 minutes, depending upon thickness of fillets. Fillets are done when they flake easily with a fork.

5 Remove from oven and serve immediately.

SERVES 4	
Per Serving:	
Calories	310
Fat	19g
Saturated Fat	4.5g
Cholesterol	80mg
Sodium	260mg
Carbohydrates	1g
Fiber	0g
Sugar	0g
Added Sugars	0g
Protein	29g

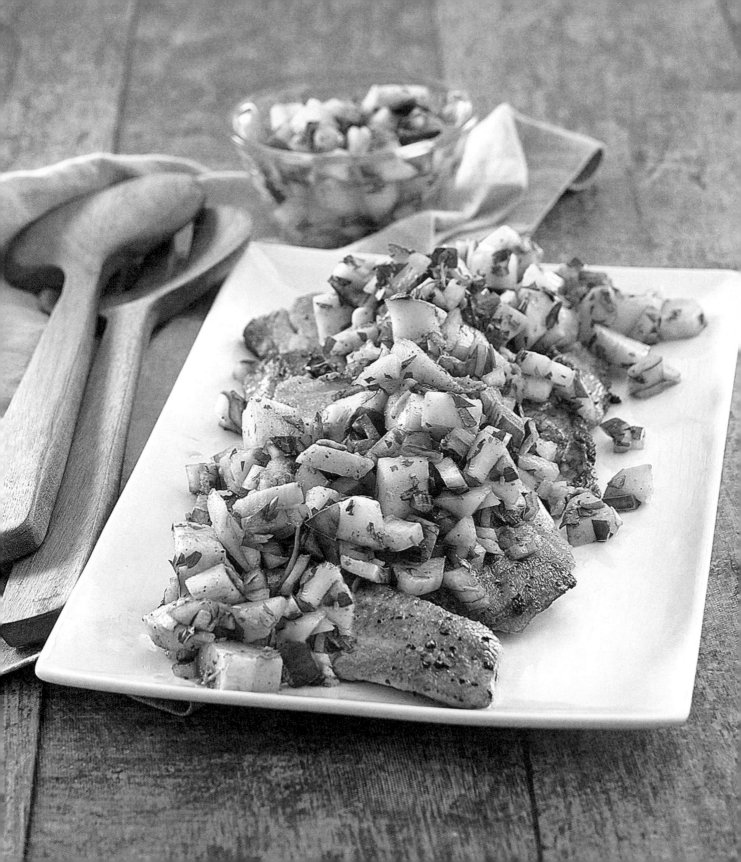

Grilled Tilapia with Peach-Mango Salsa

Sweet, salt, acid, and heat round out the flavor profile of this simple entrée. Serve it with grilled or roasted vegetables and a small portion of a whole grain like farro, quinoa, or brown rice. Or create a fish taco by wrapping the tilapia and salsa in a high-fiber tortilla.

2 tablespoons olive oil

2 tablespoons lime juice

¼ teaspoon salt

¼ teaspoon ground black pepper

1½ pounds tilapia fillets

1 cup Fresh Peach-Mango Salsa (see Chapter 9)

1 In a medium shallow dish, mix oil, lime juice, salt, and black pepper. Add tilapia and turn to coat fish with marinade.

2 Heat gas or charcoal grill or broiler to high. Spray a large piece of aluminum foil with nonstick cooking spray. Place fillets on foil and cook 7–8 minutes on each side, or until fish is tender when pierced with a fork.

3 Top each piece of fish with ¼ cup Fresh Peach-Mango Salsa. Serve.

SERVES 4	
Per Serving:	
Calories	190
Fat	4g
Saturated Fat	1g
Cholesterol	85mg
Sodium	160mg
Carbohydrates	5g
Fiber	1g
Sugar	4g
Added Sugars	0g
Protein	35g

Shrimp Creole

Per Serving:

Calories	210
Fat	3.5g
Saturated Fat	0g
Cholesterol	185mg
Sodium	650mg
Carbohydrates	14g
Fiber	4g
Sugar	8g
Added Sugars	0g
Protein	26g

This spicy and beautiful shrimp dish is made for special occasions. Serve over cooked brown rice or riced cauliflower for a lower-carb meal.

2 teaspoons canola oil

1 medium onion, peeled and thinly sliced

1 medium red bell pepper, seeded and thinly sliced

2 medium stalks celery, thinly sliced

3 medium cloves garlic, peeled and minced

2 (15-ounce) cans diced tomatoes, undrained

1 (8-ounce) can tomato sauce

⅓ cup dry white wine

½ teaspoon apple cider vinegar

2 medium bay leaves

2 teaspoons chili seasoning

1 teaspoon ground sweet paprika

½ teaspoon ground black pepper

⅛ teaspoon ground cayenne pepper

1 pound shrimp, shelled and deveined

1 In a medium sauté pan over medium heat, heat oil. Add onion, bell pepper, celery, and garlic and cook, stirring, 5 minutes.

2 Add remaining ingredients except shrimp and stir well to combine. Simmer 10 minutes, stirring frequently. Cover and reduce heat to medium-low if sauce begins to splatter.

3 Stir in shrimp and simmer 5 minutes.

4 Remove from heat and remove bay leaves from pan. Serve immediately.

Honey Dijon Tuna Salad

This salad is perfect on its own for a light lunch, but you can also turn it into a pasta salad by adding 1 cup cold cooked whole-grain pasta shells to the tuna mixture.

1 (5-ounce) can water-packed solid white tuna, drained

½ cup diced celery

¼ cup diced yellow onion

½ cup diced red bell pepper

¼ cup plain nonfat Greek yogurt

1 teaspoon Dijon mustard

1 teaspoon lemon juice

¼ teaspoon honey

2 tablespoons raisins

2 cups tightly packed mixed salad greens

SERVES 2	
Per Serving:	
Calories	150
Fat	1g
Saturated Fat	0g
Cholesterol	25mg
Sodium	310mg
Carbohydrates	18g
Fiber	4g
Sugar	12g
Added Sugars	1g
Protein	19g

1 Use a fork to flake tuna into a medium bowl. Add celery, onion, bell pepper, yogurt, mustard, lemon juice, honey, and raisins and mix well.

2 Serve over salad greens.

Baked Bread Crumb–Crusted Fish with Lemon

Lemon is the star in this easy-to-make dish. Juice, zest, and lemon slices all add bright, fresh flavor to the mild whitefish.

SERVES 6

Per Serving:

Calories	120
Fat	1.5g
Saturated Fat	0g
Cholesterol	55mg
Sodium	190mg
Carbohydrates	3g
Fiber	0g
Sugar	0g
Added Sugars	0g
Protein	22g

LEMON INFUSION

Mildly flavored fish such as catfish, cod, halibut, orange roughy, rockfish, and snapper benefit from the distinctive flavor of lemon. Adding slices of lemon to the dish allows the flavor to infuse into the fish.

2 large lemons
¼ cup dried whole-grain bread crumbs
1½ pounds halibut fillets
½ teaspoon kosher salt
¼ teaspoon ground black pepper
1 tablespoon minced fresh parsley

1 Preheat oven to 375°F. Spray a medium baking dish with nonstick cooking spray and set aside.

2 Cut one lemon into thin slices. Grate 1 tablespoon of zest from second lemon, and then squeeze juice into a small bowl.

3 In a separate small bowl, combine lemon zest and bread crumbs and stir to mix.

4 Arrange lemon slices in bottom of prepared baking dish. Dip fish pieces in lemon juice and then set on lemon slices.

5 Sprinkle bread crumb mixture evenly over fish, along with salt and black pepper. Bake until crumbs are lightly browned and fish is just opaque, approximately 13 minutes.

6 Transfer fish and lemon slices to a medium serving dish and sprinkle with parsley. Serve immediately.

Spicy Garlic Shrimp

Ready in a flash, this flavorful shrimp is fabulous served with Sautéed Spinach and Garlic (see Chapter 6) and ½ cup of your favorite whole grain such as whole-wheat or bean-based pasta, whole-grain rice, quinoa, farro, or sorghum.

1 tablespoon olive oil

10 medium cloves garlic, peeled and chopped

1 pound extra-large shrimp (approximately 26–30), shelled and deveined

¼ teaspoon kosher salt

½ teaspoon ground paprika

¼ teaspoon red pepper flakes

1 In a medium sauté pan over medium heat, heat oil. Add garlic and sauté until fragrant but not brown, approximately 30 seconds.

2 Add shrimp and salt and stir frequently until shrimp is cooked through, approximately 2 minutes.

3 Remove pan from heat and stir in paprika. Add red pepper flakes and serve.

SERVES 4

Per Serving:

Calories	140
Fat	4g
Saturated Fat	1g
Cholesterol	185mg
Sodium	210mg
Carbohydrates	3g
Fiber	0g
Sugar	0g
Added Sugars	0g
Protein	23g

Grilled Chili-Lime Shrimp

SERVES 2

Per Serving:

Calories	100
Fat	0.5g
Saturated Fat	0g
Cholesterol	185mg
Sodium	135mg
Carbohydrates	1g
Fiber	0g
Sugar	1g
Added Sugars	1g
Protein	23g

DON'T WORRY ABOUT THE SUGAR IN A MARINADE

While your instinct may be to avoid all sugar, it's really not necessary, especially in a marinade. Most of the marinade doesn't make its way through the cooking process, so you are only consuming a fraction of the sugar in the final entrée.

Made with just four simple ingredients, these flavorful grilled shrimp are delicious served as an appetizer, on top of a salad, in tacos, or with stir-fried vegetables.

¼ cup lime juice

4 teaspoons light brown sugar

½ teaspoon chili powder

8 ounces (about 12–14) shrimp, shelled with tails remaining and deveined

1 In a small bowl, whisk together lime juice, brown sugar, and chili powder.

2 Place shrimp in a large zip-top plastic bag and add lime mixture. Marinate 10 minutes on countertop.

3 Meanwhile, heat a gas or charcoal grill to high heat. Soak four wooden skewers in water 10 minutes.

4 Remove shrimp from bag and discard marinade. Thread 3–4 shrimp on each skewer.

5 Grill 2 minutes per side until shrimp are slightly pink. Serve.

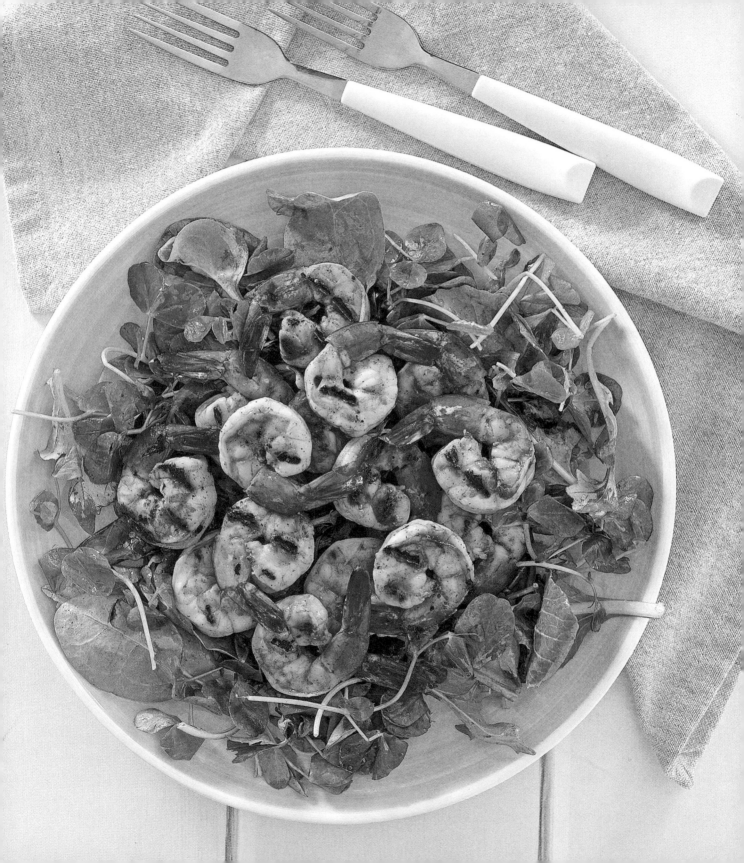

Balsamic Tuna Grain Salad

SERVES 2	
Per Serving:	
Calories	350
Fat	14g
Saturated Fat	3g
Cholesterol	40mg
Sodium	190mg
Carbohydrates	39g
Fiber	6g
Sugar	6g
Added Sugars	1g
Protein	25g

ANY WHOLE GRAIN WILL DO

This recipe is an excellent way to use up leftover grains, including any whole grain of your choosing. Try farro, wild rice, quinoa, or wheat berries.

Light and satisfying, this dish packs well for lunch on the go. It's a fabulous way to use up any leftover cooked grains.

1 cup packed cooked whole-grain sorghum

1 (5-ounce) can water-packed no-salt-added solid white tuna, drained

1 cup grape tomatoes

¼ cup diced red onion

½ medium avocado, peeled, pitted, and diced

1 tablespoon olive oil

1 tablespoon plain nonfat Greek yogurt

2 tablespoons balsamic vinegar

¾ teaspoon honey

1⁄16 teaspoon kosher salt

1⁄16 teaspoon ground black pepper

2 cups romaine lettuce, chopped

1 In a medium bowl, add sorghum, tuna, tomatoes, onion, and avocado.

2 In a small bowl mix oil, yogurt, vinegar, honey, salt, and black pepper.

3 Stir 2 tablespoons dressing into tuna mixture. Serve atop lettuce and drizzle with additional 1 teaspoon dressing. Reserve remaining dressing for another time.

CHAPTER 6

Vegetarian Mains and Sides

Vegan Lentil Sloppy Joes

Beans and legumes are an ally in lowering blood sugar, and this recipe will be on repeat once your family tries it. It's so delicious, no one will miss the meat. Serve these sloppy joes on a whole-grain or fiber-enriched bun.

1 tablespoon olive oil

½ small onion, peeled and diced small

½ medium red bell pepper, seeded and diced small

1 medium clove garlic, peeled and finely chopped

1 cup canned tomato sauce

1 tablespoon tomato paste

¼ cup no-sugar-added ketchup

2 teaspoons vegan Worcestershire sauce

½ teaspoon apple cider vinegar

½ teaspoon golden monk fruit or brown sugar–style erythritol

1 (15-ounce) can lentils, drained and rinsed

¼ teaspoon kosher salt

¼ teaspoon ground black pepper

1 In a medium nonstick skillet over medium heat, heat olive oil. Add onion, pepper, and garlic and sauté until soft, about 2–3 minutes.

2 Add remaining ingredients except lentils, salt, and black pepper and stir to combine.

3 Add lentils, salt, and pepper and bring to a gentle boil. Cook an additional 5 minutes to thicken, stirring often.

Tofu Panko Parmesan

You don't need to identify as vegetarian or vegan to benefit from more plant-based meals. Forgo the chicken Parmesan and substitute tofu instead. Eating soy foods has been shown to lower cholesterol, decrease blood glucose levels, and improve glucose tolerance in people with diabetes.

1 (14-ounce) package firm tofu

1 cup whole-wheat panko bread crumbs (see sidebar)

½ teaspoon dried oregano

¼ teaspoon garlic powder

¼ teaspoon kosher salt

1 tablespoon chopped fresh parsley

1 large egg

¾ cup low-sodium marinara sauce

½ cup shredded reduced-fat (2%) mozzarella cheese

2 tablespoons chopped fresh basil

SERVES 4	
Per Serving:	
Calories	230
Fat	9g
Saturated Fat	1.5g
Cholesterol	55mg
Sodium	270mg
Carbohydrates	22g
Fiber	4g
Sugar	3g
Added Sugars	1g
Protein	18g

1 Heat oven to 375°F. Line a medium baking sheet with foil and spray with nonstick cooking spray.

2 Drain water from tofu and blot *very well* with paper towels. Slice tofu into four even slices lengthwise so they are large, thin rectangles. Continue to blot each slice with paper towels until they are almost dry.

3 On a medium shallow plate, combine bread crumbs, oregano, garlic powder, salt, and parsley.

4 In a medium wide-bottomed bowl, beat egg. Dip each tofu slice into egg and then into bread crumb mixture. Place tofu slices onto baking sheet and spray tops with nonstick cooking spray.

5 Bake 10 minutes until lightly browned. Add 2–3 tablespoons sauce to each piece and top with approximately 2 tablespoons mozzarella. Bake an additional 5 minutes until cheese melts.

6 Remove from oven and garnish with basil.

HOW TO MAKE YOUR OWN BREAD CRUMBS

Whole-wheat panko bread crumbs are sometimes difficult to find. Make your own by placing high-fiber bread that's on the way to stale in a food processor or blender. Spread out the crumbs on a medium foil-lined baking sheet and toast or bake at 350°F until crispy. One slice of "light" bread yields ⅓–½ cup crumbs.

Caramelized Onions

SERVES 4

Per Serving (¼ cup):

Calories	80
Fat	3.5g
Saturated Fat	0.5g
Cholesterol	0mg
Sodium	0mg
Carbohydrates	11g
Fiber	2g
Sugar	5g
Added Sugars	0g
Protein	1g

TIMESAVING TIP

This recipe can be made ahead of time and kept on hand in a small glass jar for 3–5 days to use as a condiment and add flavor to many dishes. Caramelized onions are wonderful on everything from sandwiches to salads and as a garnish for roasts and stews.

Onions go well on almost everything. Having them ready ahead of time for salads, sandwiches, burgers, or wraps makes adding more vegetables to your diet easy. High in vitamin C, onions are a good source of dietary fiber and folic acid and can help protect against heart disease.

3 large Vidalia or other sweet onions, peeled and sliced ⅛" thick

1 tablespoon olive oil

Place onions in a large sauté pan with oil. Over very low heat, sauté 20 minutes, or until onions are browned but not burned. Serve or refrigerate for later.

Sautéed Spinach and Garlic

A bed of sautéed spinach is a terrific low-carb base for so many meat, fish, poultry, and vegetarian entrees. Keep some on hand in the refrigerator to add to tortilla pizzas, wraps, sandwiches, and omelets.

1 tablespoon extra-virgin olive oil

1 tablespoon chopped garlic

1 pound baby spinach

½ teaspoon kosher salt

⅛ teaspoon ground black pepper

1 Heat a large pot over medium-high heat. Once hot, add oil and then garlic and sauté 20 seconds.

2 Add spinach and use tongs to turn leaves, lifting garlic off the bottom so it doesn't burn.

3 Stir spinach until wilted. Fold in salt and black pepper. Serve.

SERVES 4	
Per Serving (½ cup):	
Calories	60
Fat	3.5g
Saturated Fat	0.5g
Cholesterol	0mg
Sodium	230mg
Carbohydrates	5g
Fiber	3g
Sugar	0g
Added Sugars	0g
Protein	3g

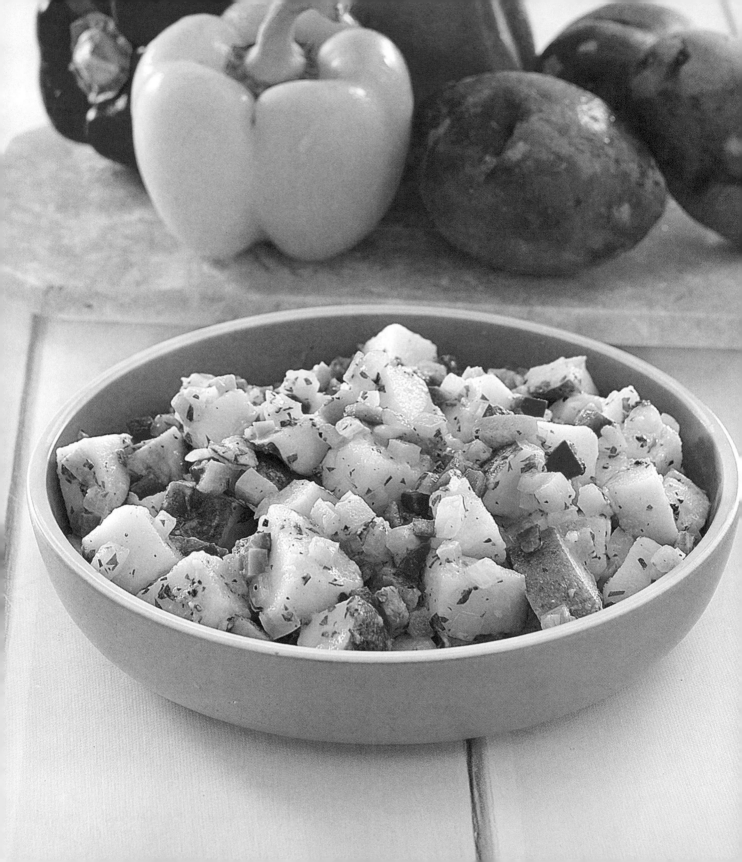

Tricolor Pepper Potato Salad

This is not your classic mayonnaise-laden potato salad. With added vegetables and an olive oil and vinegar base, this dish gives you a nutrient-rich, heart-healthy party dish that's pretty too.

2 pounds red potatoes, chopped into ½" pieces

1½ teaspoons salt, divided

1 tablespoon apple cider vinegar

⅓ cup plus 1 tablespoon extra-virgin olive oil, divided

½ large yellow onion, peeled and diced

½ medium yellow bell pepper, seeded and chopped

½ medium orange bell pepper, seeded and chopped

½ medium red bell pepper, seeded and chopped

3 tablespoons dry white wine

2 tablespoons low-sodium vegetable broth

1½ tablespoons lemon juice

½ teaspoon minced garlic

½ teaspoon Dijon mustard

½ teaspoon ground black pepper

3 tablespoons chopped fresh parsley

1. Place potatoes in a large pot and cover with water. Add 1 teaspoon salt and bring to a boil. Simmer until just slightly underdone, approximately 15 minutes.
2. Remove potatoes from pot with slotted spoon and place in a large bowl. Add vinegar and stir. Set aside.
3. Meanwhile, heat 1 tablespoon oil in a medium sauté pan over medium-high heat. Add onion and sauté 3 minutes, then add bell peppers. Reduce heat to medium and gently sauté approximately 20 minutes until peppers are soft. During the last few minutes, turn heat to medium-high to allow onions and peppers to brown.
4. While vegetables are cooking, in a medium bowl, combine wine, broth, lemon juice, garlic, mustard, remaining ½ teaspoon salt, and black pepper. Slowly whisk in remaining ⅓ cup oil until combined; set aside.
5. Add vegetables to potatoes and slowly add dressing while gently stirring. Add parsley and serve warm if desired. It's even more delicious if flavors are allowed to develop in refrigerator overnight.

SERVES 12

Per Serving (½ cup):

Calories	130
Fat	8g
Saturated Fat	1.5g
Cholesterol	0mg
Sodium	170mg
Carbohydrates	14g
Fiber	2g
Sugar	2g
Added Sugars	0g
Protein	2g

EMBRACE POTATOES

Potatoes are not taboo with pre-diabetes; in fact, they contain important nutrients like potassium and vitamin C. A little-known secret is that when potatoes are cooked and then cooled as in potato salad, they form resistant starch that slows digestion and blunts a rise in blood sugar.

Broccoli Rabe with Pine Nuts

Resembling a cross between broccoli and spinach, broccoli rabe is full of vitamins A, C, and K, and also packs in minerals like calcium, folate, and iron. Its antioxidants and phytochemicals can help combat heart disease and cancer.

Per Serving:

Calories	90
Fat	6g
Saturated Fat	1g
Cholesterol	0mg
Sodium	180mg
Carbohydrates	6g
Fiber	3g
Sugar	2g
Added Sugars	0g
Protein	4g

PREVENTING BITTER BROCCOLI RABE

Broccoli rabe can have a bitter taste once cooked. Rather than add extra salt to offset bitterness, this recipe calls for blanching 2 minutes, which helps reduce bitterness. Blanching should be done as quickly as possible by starting with water at full rolling boil, then removing after 2 minutes of boiling. If allowed to cook too long, the boiling process will reduce the amount of water-soluble nutrients found in the vegetables.

12 ounces broccoli rabe

1 tablespoon olive oil

4 medium cloves garlic, peeled and chopped

¼ cup chopped sun-dried tomatoes

2 tablespoons pine nuts

¼ teaspoon salt

¼ teaspoon red pepper flakes

1 Rinse broccoli rabe well and trim stems. Loosely chop leafy parts and remaining stems, then blanch in 2 quarts boiling water for 2 minutes. Drain well.

2 In a large skillet over medium heat, heat oil. Add garlic and sauté 1–2 minutes. Add blanched broccoli rabe. Toss garlic and broccoli rabe together well, so that oil and garlic are mixed evenly.

3 Add remaining ingredients and cook an additional 2–3 minutes until tender. Serve.

Cranberry Orange Ginger Relish

This no-cook festive recipe is so versatile and a nutritious alternative to sugar-laden cranberry sauce. My secret ingredient is a bit of ground ginger, which adds a pop of flavor. Use the leftovers on pancakes, waffles, cottage cheese, yogurt, turkey sandwiches, and more.

1 medium apple such as Gala, Fuji, Honeycrisp, cored and cut into cubes

1 large clementine/mandarin, peeled and quartered

2 cups fresh cranberries

1 teaspoon clementine/mandarin zest

3 tablespoons spoonable stevia, monk fruit, or erythritol

⅛ teaspoon ground ginger

2 ounces (about ½ cup) walnuts, chopped

1 In a blender or food processor, pulse apple gently until you have small pieces (don't purée) and transfer to a medium bowl.

2 Using the same pulsing method, process clementine/mandarin and transfer to same bowl. Next process cranberries in two batches and transfer to bowl.

3 Add zest, stevia, and ginger and stir to combine.

4 Add walnuts, stir, cover, and refrigerate at least 2 hours to let flavors develop before serving

SERVES 6

Per Serving (½ cup):

Calories	100
Fat	6g
Saturated Fat	0.5g
Cholesterol	0mg
Sodium	0mg
Carbohydrates	11g
Fiber	3g
Sugar	5g
Added Sugars	0g
Protein	2g

HOW TO TOAST WALNUTS

Toasting the walnuts first is not necessary but certainly adds dimension to the flavors of the relish. Place the nuts on aluminum foil and toast for 2–3 minutes making sure not to burn them. Let cool for a couple of minutes before adding them to the fruit. You can also toast them in a dry sauté pan for a few minutes over medium heat.

Cauliflower Latkes

SERVES 12

Per Serving (1 pancake):

Calories	70
Fat	4g
Saturated Fat	1.5g
Cholesterol	35mg
Sodium	105mg
Carbohydrates	4g
Fiber	1g
Sugar	1g
Added Sugars	0g
Protein	4g

RICED CAULIFLOWER

You can find riced cauliflower premade in the produce or freezer sections of the supermarket. Chopped cauliflower crumbles are not small enough to make these pancakes. If purchasing these crumbles, toss them in the blender and pulse until you have the consistency of rice, the smaller the better to make these stick together. To make your own, add about ½ head of cauliflower broken in pieces to a blender or food processor and gently pulse until you have the consistency of rice.

Cauliflower Latkes are a vegetable-packed tasty alternative to traditional potato latkes. They're low in carbohydrates and sautéed in just a little oil versus deep-fried. Serve with sour cream, Greek yogurt, tzatziki, or cottage cheese. For an extra kick, add some sriracha, red pepper flakes, or smoked paprika.

1 (16-ounce) package riced cauliflower (approximately 4 cups)

2 large eggs

1 large egg white or 3 tablespoons liquid egg whites

¼ teaspoon garlic powder

½ teaspoon kosher salt

½ teaspoon ground black pepper

½ cup shredded reduced-fat (2%) Cheddar or Mexican blend cheese

3 tablespoons chopped scallion

¼ cup white whole-wheat flour

2 tablespoons extra-virgin olive oil, divided

1 In a large bowl, combine all ingredients except oil and mix well.

2 Heat a large sauté pan over medium to medium-high heat and add 2 teaspoons oil.

3 Pack a ¼-cup measuring cup with cauliflower mixture, add to pan, and gently flatten. (Cook four pancakes at a time in pan.) Sauté 2–3 minutes until bottom is browned and holding together. Gently flip pancakes and cook second side 2 minutes or until nicely browned.

4 Line a medium plate with paper towels. Remove pancakes from pan and place on plate to drain.

5 Repeat the process two more times for a total of twelve pancakes.

Zucchini au Gratin Cups

Though typically baked in a casserole, preparing this flavorful side dish in muffin tins makes portion control so easy and fun. Plus, they cook much faster!

2 teaspoons olive oil

2 medium zucchini, sliced very thin

4 large fresh basil leaves, chopped

2 teaspoons chopped fresh parsley

4 ounces (about 1 cup) shredded reduced-fat (2%) mozzarella or Italian blend cheese

2 tablespoons grated Parmesan cheese

¼ cup whole-grain seasoned bread crumbs

1 Preheat oven to 350°F. Spray a twelve-cup muffin tin with olive oil spray.

2 In a large bowl, combine oil and zucchini, working through with your hands to make sure oil is evenly distributed.

3 Add basil, parsley, mozzarella, and Parmesan and combine well.

4 Divide mixture among muffin cups and top with bread crumbs. Cover with foil and bake 20 minutes.

5 Remove foil and continue cooking approximately 10 more minutes until cheese is melted and bread crumbs are nicely browned. Serve.

SERVES 12	
Per Serving:	
Calories	50
Fat	3g
Saturated Fat	1.5g
Cholesterol	5mg
Sodium	130mg
Carbohydrates	3g
Fiber	0g
Sugar	1g
Added Sugars	0g
Protein	4g

Brussels Sprouts Hash with Caramelized Shallots

SERVES 4

Per Serving:

Calories	150
Fat	11g
Saturated Fat	2g
Cholesterol	0mg
Sodium	90mg
Carbohydrates	13g
Fiber	4g
Sugar	3g
Added Sugars	0g
Protein	4g

Brussels sprouts are high in antioxidants, fiber, and vitamins C, K, and B. They are delicious roasted, and the balsamic vinegar adds just the right amount of acidity and sweetness. Pair them with any protein, add to a grain bowl, or use in your favorite salad.

1 pound Brussels sprouts, stems trimmed, halved lengthwise

2 medium shallots, peeled and thinly sliced

3 tablespoons olive oil

¼ teaspoon kosher salt

⅛ teaspoon ground black pepper

3 tablespoons balsamic vinegar

1 Preheat oven to 400°F.
2 Place Brussels sprouts and shallots in a medium shallow baking dish. Coat Brussels sprouts with oil and season with salt and black pepper.
3 Bake 20 minutes, stirring halfway through cooking time. Remove dish from oven and drizzle vinegar evenly over Brussels sprouts. Return dish to oven to bake 3–4 more minutes, taking care not to burn shallots. Serve.

Roasted Garlic Mashed Potatoes

Combining cauliflower with potatoes is an excellent way to pump up your vegetable consumption while increasing the portion size of a favorite comfort food. To make the process even easier, use frozen riced cauliflower cooked in the microwave.

4 cloves dry-roasted garlic (see sidebar in recipe for Garlic and Feta Cheese Spread in Chapter 3) or 1 teaspoon roasted garlic paste

1 small onion, peeled and chopped

12 ounces potatoes, peeled and boiled until soft

2 cups cauliflower florets, steamed and drained

¼ cup buttermilk

2 tablespoons low-fat cottage cheese

2 teaspoons unsalted butter

½ teaspoon kosher salt

¼ teaspoon ground black pepper

Place all ingredients into a food processor. Pulse until fluffy. Serve.

SERVES 4	
Per Serving:	
Calories	160
Fat	6g
Saturated Fat	4g
Cholesterol	15mg
Sodium	210mg
Carbohydrates	24g
Fiber	3g
Sugar	4g
Added Sugars	0g
Protein	4g

GRAVY SUBSTITUTE

Instead of using gravy, sprinkle crumbled bleu cheese or grated Parmesan over these mashed potatoes.

Parmesan-Roasted Campari Tomatoes

SERVES 8

Per Serving (2 tomato halves):

Calories	35
Fat	2g
Saturated Fat	0.5g
Cholesterol	0mg
Sodium	35mg
Carbohydrates	4g
Fiber	1g
Sugar	2g
Added Sugars	0g
Protein	2g

WHAT ARE CAMPARI TOMATOES?

Campari is a type of tomato known for its juiciness, high-sugar level, low acidity, and lack of mealiness. Deeper red and larger than a cherry tomato, but smaller and rounder than a plum tomato, Camparis are a beautiful ruby red and perfectly sized to cut in half for roasting.

A simple summer side dish or salad topper, these roasted tomatoes elevate the flavor of so many dishes. Add to pasta, a grain bowl, or grilled chicken, fish, or meat. Pair with an omelet for breakfast to start your day with extra vegetables.

8 Campari tomatoes, halved

2 tablespoons grated Parmesan cheese

½ teaspoon dried oregano

⅛ teaspoon ground black pepper

2 teaspoons extra-virgin olive oil

⅛ teaspoon red pepper flakes

1 tablespoon chopped fresh basil, for garnish

1 Preheat oven to 400°F.
2 Place tomatoes cut side up on a medium baking sheet covered with nonstick foil or aluminum foil sprayed with nonstick cooking spray.
3 Sprinkle Parmesan, oregano, and black pepper evenly over tomatoes. Carefully drizzle with oil and sprinkle with red pepper flakes.
4 Roast long enough for cheese to melt and lightly brown but before tomatoes become mushy, approximately 10–15 minutes. Sprinkle basil on top and serve.

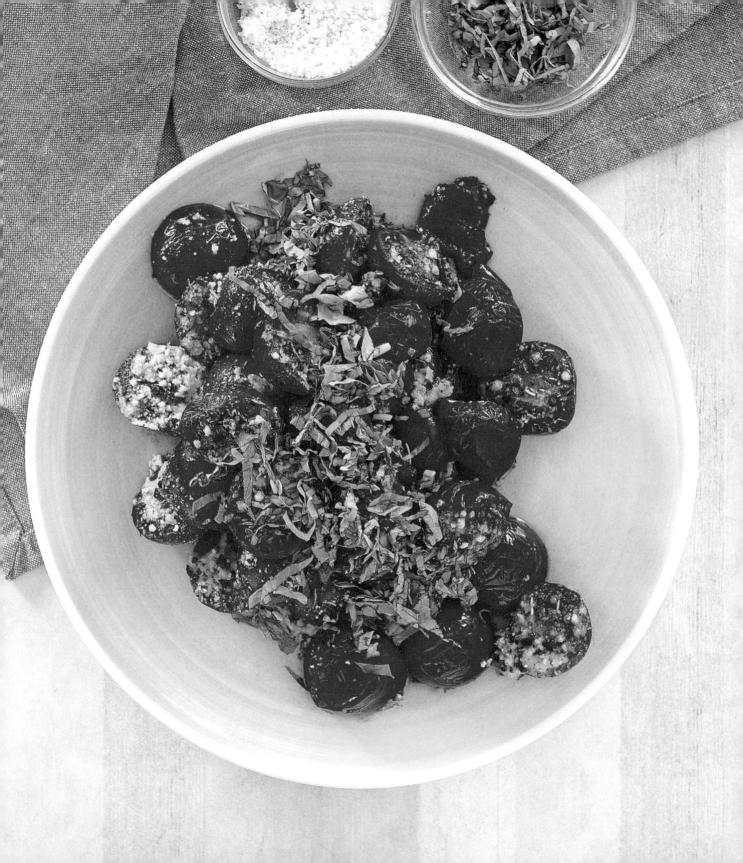

Spaghetti Squash Hash

Hash browns don't have to be made from potatoes. Spaghetti squash brings a new and different flavor to a cheesy hash that complements eggs, a tofu scramble, or any protein for a unique low-carb side dish. Switch up the cheese type to adjust the flavor profile from mild to spicy.

HOW TO COOK SPAGHETTI SQUASH

Roasting spaghetti squash can take 45–60 minutes in the oven depending on the size of the squash. To speed up the process, use a pressure cooker and you will have a fully cooked squash in about 15 minutes.

2 cups cooked spaghetti squash

¼ cup diced yellow onion

1 large egg

¼ teaspoon garlic powder

¼ teaspoon kosher salt

⅛ teaspoon ground black pepper

¼ cup plus 2 tablespoons shredded reduced-fat (2%) Mexican cheese, divided

1 Spray a medium nonstick sauté pan with nonstick cooking spray and heat over medium-high heat. Squeeze out extra moisture from spaghetti squash with cheesecloth or paper towels.

2 In a medium bowl, add squash, onion, egg, garlic powder, salt, and black pepper, mixing to combine.

3 Add mixture to pan, flatten it out, and sprinkle with ¼ cup shredded cheese. Let cook undisturbed approximately 5 minutes. Then stir occasionally an additional 10 minutes until most of the moisture is removed and squash is lightly browned.

4 Divide into two servings and top each with 1 tablespoon remaining shredded cheese.

Roasted Cabbage Steaks

Cabbage steaks are a great addition to salads, sandwiches, wraps, tacos, and much more. Use them as a base for grilled salmon, chicken, or steak and use whatever spices you prefer to match the flavor of the accompanying protein.

1 medium (about 1½–2 pounds) red or green cabbage
½ teaspoon kosher salt
¼ teaspoon ground black pepper
1 teaspoon ground paprika

1 Preheat oven to 425°F. Line two medium baking sheets with silicone liners or spray generously with nonstick cooking spray.

2 Cut bottom core off cabbage to make a flat surface and clear away any wilted or damaged leaves. Slice it from top to bottom in ¼" slices.

3 Spread slices out on baking sheets and spray tops with nonstick cooking spray. Sprinkle with salt, black pepper, and paprika.

4 Roast 12 minutes, then switch position of trays in oven. Continue to cook an additional 10–12 minutes until cabbage is easily pierced with a fork and edges have browned. Serve.

SERVES 4	
Per Serving:	
Calories	90
Fat	4g
Saturated Fat	0.5g
Cholesterol	0mg
Sodium	180mg
Carbohydrates	14g
Fiber	6g
Sugar	7g
Added Sugars	0g
Protein	3g

Tofu Pesto Shirataki

Per Serving:

Calories	340
Fat	26g
Saturated Fat	5g
Cholesterol	10mg
Sodium	700mg
Carbohydrates	9g
Fiber	5.5g
Sugar	1g
Added Sugars	0g
Protein	23g

WHAT ARE SHIRATAKI-STYLE NOODLES?

Those looking for low-carb pasta alternatives have an option in shirataki noodles. Shirataki, meaning "white waterfall" in Japanese, is a traditional Japanese noodle made with an Asian yam called konjac (or konnyaku). If you have never prepared shirataki, it's precooked. You just drain the water out of the package, rinse, microwave briefly and pat noodles dry. Now you are ready to add them to any dish.

Would you love to enjoy a satisfying dish with the pasta portion containing only 10–20 calories per serving? Shirataki noodles are the base for this meatless meal that's a simple addition to your vegetarian rotation. Garnish the noodles with some fresh parsley or basil.

6 ounces firm or extra-firm tofu

⅛ teaspoon salt

⅛ teaspoon ground black pepper

2 teaspoons extra-virgin olive oil

1 bag tofu shirataki noodles, fettuccine style

1 tablespoon jarred pesto

1 tablespoon grated Parmesan cheese

1 Drain tofu and press with paper towels or a tofu press until liquid is removed. Cut into approximately sixteen cubes and blot dry again with paper towels. Season top and bottom sides of tofu cubes with salt and black pepper.

2 Heat a medium sauté pan over medium heat and add oil. Add tofu cubes and sauté, turning every 2 minutes until lightly browned on three or four sides.

3 Meanwhile, drain shirataki noodles and prepare according to the package directions. Dry thoroughly.

4 When tofu is done, add noodles and pesto to pan. Heat and stir 5 minutes. Transfer to a medium plate and garnish with Parmesan. Serve.

Healthy Onion Rings

These onion rings have a fraction of the fat of standard fast-food fare and are delightfully crispy thanks to the whole-grain cereal. Experiment with seasonings to suit your taste. Try a little cayenne pepper to make them spicy or perhaps a sprinkle of Parmesan or garlic powder.

½ cup white whole-wheat flour

½ cup plain nonfat Greek yogurt

½ cup high-fiber cereal, such as Fiber One, ground into a powder

1 medium yellow onion, peeled and sliced into ¼"-thick rings

¼ teaspoon kosher salt

¼ teaspoon ground black pepper

1 Preheat oven to 350°F. Prepare a medium baking sheet with non-stick cooking spray or a silicone liner and set aside.

2 Place flour in one medium shallow dish, the yogurt in a separate medium dish, and the cereal crumbs in a third.

3 Dredge onion slices first in flour; shake off any excess. Next dip onions in yogurt and then dredge through cereal crumbs.

4 Arrange onion rings on prepared baking sheet and spray lightly with nonstick cooking spray. Bake on top rack 20 minutes.

5 Season with salt and black pepper and serve.

SERVES 4	
Per Serving:	
Calories	120
Fat	3g
Saturated Fat	0g
Cholesterol	0mg
Sodium	105mg
Carbohydrates	22g
Fiber	6g
Sugar	2g
Added Sugars	0g
Protein	6g

Cauliflower and Mushroom Taco Filling

SERVES 4	
Per Serving:	
Calories	100
Fat	4g
Saturated Fat	0.5g
Cholesterol	0mg
Sodium	130mg
Carbohydrates	12g
Fiber	4g
Sugar	5g
Added Sugars	0g
Protein	5g

This vegetarian filling can be wrapped in tortillas or lettuce wraps, scooped atop a salad, or served on its own as a delicious side dish. If you like, add beans, cheese, salsa, and avocado for a delicious meatless meal.

4 cups frozen riced cauliflower

1 tablespoon olive oil

4 cups chopped baby bella mushrooms

1 cup chopped white onion

½ tablespoon chili powder

½ tablespoon ground cumin

¼ teaspoon kosher salt

1 Place cauliflower rice in a large microwave-safe baking dish and microwave on high 4 minutes. Set aside.

2 Meanwhile, in a large skillet over medium heat, heat oil 30 seconds. Add mushrooms and onion and sauté until lightly browned, about 5 minutes.

3 Add cauliflower, chili powder, and cumin to skillet. Stir to distribute spices. Cook, stirring occasionally, 5 minutes until lightly browned and tender and liquid has absorbed. Serve.

Peppery Swiss Chard

Rainbow chard is so beautiful and adds personality to any plate. Red pepper flakes give it a little kick and decreases the need for salt.

1 bunch fresh Swiss chard (about 12 ounces trimmed)

2 teaspoons olive oil

2 medium cloves garlic, peeled and thinly sliced

¼ teaspoon red pepper flakes

⅛ teaspoon ground black pepper

1 Trim each Swiss chard by removing most of each stalk, leaving just 1"–2" of stalk beneath leafy portion. Chop into 2" pieces and set aside.

2 In a medium sauté pan over medium heat, heat oil. Add garlic and sauté 1 minute, taking care not to burn.

3 Add Swiss chard and sauté 6–8 minutes, turning frequently and keeping an eye on the garlic.

4 Remove from heat and stir in red pepper flakes. Season with black pepper. Serve immediately.

SERVES 4	
Per Serving:	
Calories	40
Fat	2.5g
Saturated Fat	0g
Cholesterol	0mg
Sodium	180mg
Carbohydrates	4g
Fiber	1g
Sugar	1g
Added Sugars	0g
Protein	2g

SWISS CHARD FACTS

Swiss chard is a dark, leafy green with colorful stalks akin to celery. It has a somewhat bitter taste that mellows with cooking and is particularly well suited to sautéing with a little olive oil and garlic. Swiss chard is an excellent source of vitamins A, C, and K, manganese, potassium, iron, and fiber, and contains antioxidants linked to the prevention of cancer and cardiovascular disease.

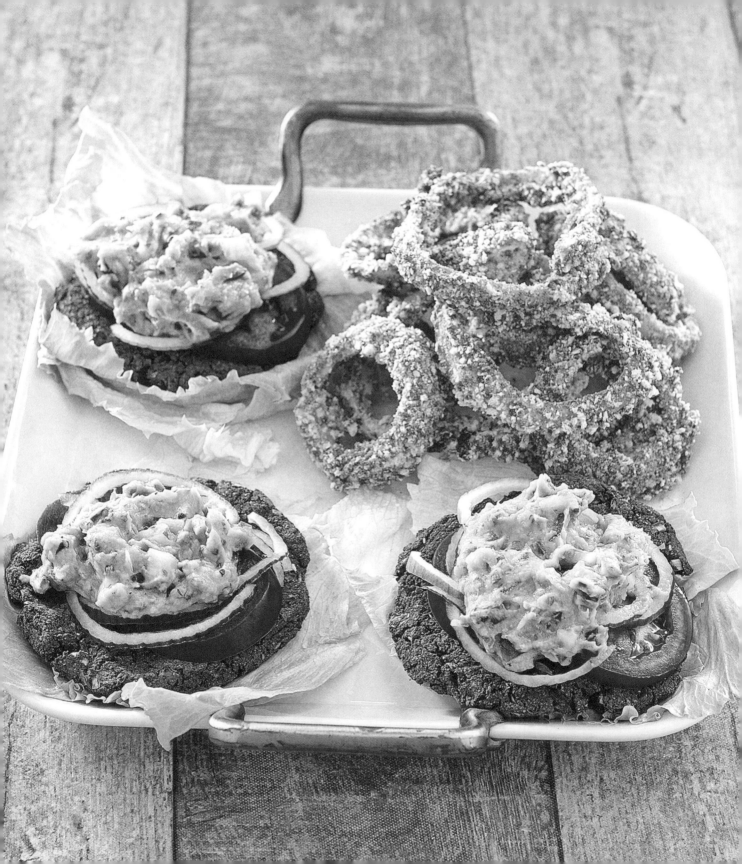

Black Bean Burgers

Southwestern flavor in a hearty, fiber-packed vegetable burger. Garnish with the Fresh Baja Guacamole in Chapter 3 or use these as the meatless protein in a taco salad. Pair it with the Healthy Onion Rings in this chapter for a full meal!

2 (15-ounce) cans low-sodium black beans, drained and rinsed

1 medium shallot, peeled and minced

3 medium cloves garlic, peeled and minced

1 medium red bell pepper, seeded and chopped

¼ cup chopped fresh cilantro

1 tablespoon lime juice

2 teaspoons chili seasoning

¼ teaspoon ground black pepper

½ cup Homemade High-Fiber Bread Crumbs (see Chapter 9)

SERVES 6	
Per Serving:	
Calories	130
Fat	0g
Saturated Fat	0g
Cholesterol	0mg
Sodium	200mg
Carbohydrates	26g
Fiber	10g
Sugar	2g
Added Sugars	0g
Protein	8g

1 Preheat oven to 425°F. Line a medium baking sheet with nonstick foil and spray lightly with nonstick cooking spray. Set aside.

2 Place beans into a food processor and purée until smooth.

3 Transfer the beans to a large mixing bowl, add remaining ingredients, and mix together using your hands. Form into six patties.

4 Place patties on prepared baking sheet. Place baking sheet on middle rack of oven and bake 10 minutes.

5 Remove from oven, gently flip, and return patties to oven. Bake an additional 5 minutes.

6 Remove from oven and serve immediately.

Baked Falafel

Though they're usually fried, baking falafel allows the flavors to shine. These are delicious in a high-fiber wrap or whole-wheat pita with hummus, tahini, or tzatziki and chopped tomatoes, cucumbers, lettuce, and fresh herbs.

1 (15-ounce) can low-sodium chickpeas, drained and rinsed

¼ medium onion, peeled and chopped (about ¼ cup)

1 large clove garlic, peeled

3 tablespoons chopped fresh parsley

½ teaspoon ground cumin

⅛ teaspoon ground cayenne pepper

½ teaspoon kosher salt

¼ teaspoon ground black pepper

1½ tablespoons crushed high-fiber cereal, such as Fiber One

¾ teaspoon baking powder

1 In a food processor, add chickpeas, onion, garlic, parsley, cumin, cayenne, salt, and black pepper. Blend until you have a coarse, even texture, scrape down the sides if needed.

2 Place mixture in a medium bowl and stir in cereal and baking powder. Cover and refrigerate about 1 hour.

3 Preheat oven to 400°F. Spray a medium baking sheet with non-stick cooking spray.

4 Form mixture into twelve balls and place on baking sheet. Coat tops of balls with nonstick cooking spray.

5 Bake 12 minutes, then turn balls over and coat other side with nonstick cooking spray. Bake 12 more minutes. Serve.

Mashed Cauliflower

If you are looking for a low-carb alternative to mashed potatoes, this is it. The olive oil adds heart-healthy fat instead of the usual butter and cream. Make batches of this cauliflower to keep on hand to pair with any dish.

4 cups cauliflower florets

2 tablespoons olive oil

1 tablespoon chopped fresh chives

½ teaspoon kosher salt

¼ teaspoon ground black pepper

1 Place cauliflower in a large pot of boiling water and cook 10 minutes. Drain well, reserving ¼ cup cooking liquid.

2 Place cauliflower into a blender or food processor with oil and reserved cooking liquid. Purée until smooth. Add chives and season with salt and black pepper. Serve.

SERVES 4	
Per Serving:	
Calories	90
Fat	7g
Saturated Fat	1.5g
Cholesterol	0mg
Sodium	170mg
Carbohydrates	5g
Fiber	2g
Sugar	2g
Added Sugars	0g
Protein	2g

Zucchini Cakes

SERVES 4

Per Serving:

Calories	60
Fat	1.5g
Saturated Fat	0g
Cholesterol	0mg
Sodium	330mg
Carbohydrates	12g
Fiber	5g
Sugar	4g
Added Sugars	1g
Protein	3g

These scrumptious oven-baked patties are a perfect way to use some of your garden surplus. Garnish with homemade horseradish sauce or tzatziki. Substitute your favorite seasoning blend for the all-purpose seasoning to change things up.

1 medium zucchini, shredded

1 small red onion, peeled and finely diced

1 large egg white

¾ cup Homemade High-Fiber Bread Crumbs (see Chapter 9)

2 teaspoons all-purpose seasoning

1 Preheat oven to 400°F. Line a medium baking sheet with nonstick aluminum foil and spray lightly with nonstick cooking spray; set aside.

2 Press shredded zucchini gently between paper towels to absorb excess liquid.

3 In a large bowl, combine zucchini, onion, egg white, Homemade High-Fiber Bread Crumbs, and all-purpose seasoning. Mix well. Shape mixture into four patties and place on prepared baking sheet.

4 Place baking sheet on middle rack in oven and bake 10 minutes. Very gently flip patties and return to oven to bake another 10 minutes.

5 Remove from oven and serve immediately.

Egg Salad Sandwiches with Radish and Cilantro

Creamy eggs contrast with the spicy bite of the radish, pungent cilantro, and a subtle rice vinegar tang. It's a seemingly incongruous combination of flavors that works so well together.

6 large hard-boiled eggs, diced

1 cup shredded radish

¼ cup chopped fresh cilantro

1 tablespoon olive oil

1 tablespoon unflavored rice vinegar

¼ teaspoon ground black pepper

2 cups fresh arugula

8 slices high-fiber, light whole-grain bread (40–50 calories)

SERVES 4	
Per Serving:	
Calories	230
Fat	13g
Saturated Fat	3g
Cholesterol	280mg
Sodium	350mg
Carbohydrates	27g
Fiber	14g
Sugar	3g
Added Sugars	0g
Protein	14g

1 In a medium bowl, add egg, radish, cilantro, oil, vinegar, and black pepper and stir well to combine.
2 Assemble sandwiches by dividing the arugula and egg salad evenly between four slices of bread. Top each with another slice. Serve immediately.

Peanut Butter and Banana "Sushi"

Elvis was definitely onto something with his favorite flavor combo: PB and banana rocks! This plant-based breakfast, lunch, or snack is super easy and fun for kids and adults alike.

SERVES 1	
Per Serving:	
Calories	270
Fat	4g
Saturated Fat	0g
Cholesterol	0mg
Sodium	370mg
Carbohydrates	57g
Fiber	16g
Sugar	16g
Added Sugars	0g
Protein	16g

3 tablespoons powdered peanut butter

1 tablespoon water

1 high protein, high-fiber flatbread (approximately 100 calories)

1 medium ripe banana, peeled

¼ teaspoon ground cinnamon

1 In a small bowl, combine powdered peanut butter and water, stirring and adding water by the ¼ teaspoon until desired consistency is reached.

2 Spread peanut butter down middle of flatbread, reserving about 1 teaspoon.

3 Place banana on top of peanut butter and roll up flatbread. Spread remaining 1 teaspoon peanut butter on outer edge of flatbread to create a seal.

4 Slice into pieces resembling a sushi roll. Sprinkle with cinnamon and serve.

VARIATIONS

For a creamier texture, stir the powdered peanut butter with unsweetened almond, cashew, or coconut milk instead of water for only a few extra calories. And, if you are a PB and J fanatic, try 100 percent grape juice as the mixer instead of water. You'll have a built-in jelly flavor without any added sugar.

Vegan Meat Sauce over Chickpea Pasta

This plant-based dish is also gluten-free and super easy to make. It's likely to fool picky eaters and meat lovers alike. Garnish this dish with fresh parsley or basil.

8 ounces dry chickpea spaghetti

8 ounces white mushrooms, thinly sliced

2 cups frozen meatless crumbles

3 cups low-sodium marinara sauce

¼ teaspoon garlic powder

⅛ teaspoon ground black pepper

⅛ teaspoon red pepper flakes

1 In a medium pot, bring water to a boil and cook spaghetti according to package directions.

2 Meanwhile, heat a large saucepan sprayed with olive oil spray over medium-high heat. Add mushrooms and sauté 2–3 minutes.

3 Add meatless crumbles and cook 4–5 minutes, allowing them to brown and water to evaporate.

4 Add sauce, garlic powder, black pepper, and red pepper flakes. Stir and heat 2 minutes.

5 To serve, add 1 cup pasta and 1 cup sauce to each of four medium bowls and serve.

SERVES 4	
Per Serving:	
Calories	390
Fat	7g
Saturated Fat	0g
Cholesterol	5mg
Sodium	330mg
Carbohydrates	58g
Fiber	8g
Sugar	13g
Added Sugars	4g
Protein	28g

Vegetable Tortilla Pizza

SERVES 1	
Per Serving:	
Calories	200
Fat	11g
Saturated Fat	4g
Cholesterol	15mg
Sodium	550mg
Carbohydrates	27g
Fiber	17g
Sugar	4g
Added Sugars	1g
Protein	14g

A fabulous quick lunch, this crispy version of homemade pizza never gets boring because you can add an endless variety of vegetables and seasonings.

1 (8") high-fiber, low-carb flour tortilla

3 tablespoons low-sodium marinara sauce

¼ cup roasted vegetables such as onions, peppers, mushrooms

¼ cup shredded reduced-fat (2%) mozzarella cheese

¼ teaspoon dried oregano

⅛ teaspoon red pepper flakes

1 Toast tortilla about 3 minutes directly on rack in a toaster oven or oven.

2 Spread sauce over tortilla and top with vegetables, cheese, oregano, and red pepper flakes.

3 Put back on toaster rack another 3 minutes or until cheese is melted. Slice into six pieces and serve.

Diner-Style Home Fries

Tender, seasoned potatoes sautéed with onion and bell pepper make the most delicious side dish at breakfast. Enjoy leftovers later in the day!

4 medium potatoes, cut into ½" cubes

2 teaspoons olive oil, divided

1 medium onion, peeled and diced

1 medium red bell pepper, seeded and diced

1 tablespoon tomato paste

2 teaspoons ground sweet paprika

½ teaspoon dried thyme

½ teaspoon garlic powder

½ teaspoon ground rosemary

¼ teaspoon kosher salt

¼ teaspoon ground black pepper

1 Place potatoes into a medium microwave-safe bowl and cover with plastic wrap. Microwave 7 minutes.

2 While potatoes are cooking, heat 1 teaspoon oil in a medium nonstick skillet over medium-high heat. Add onion and bell pepper and cook, stirring, 7 minutes.

3 Add cooked potatoes to skillet, along with tomato paste, paprika, thyme, garlic powder, rosemary, salt, and black pepper. Drizzle with remaining 1 teaspoon oil. Stir to combine, then cook, stirring, another 5 minutes. Remove from heat and serve.

SERVES 6

Per Serving:

Calories	90
Fat	2g
Saturated Fat	0g
Cholesterol	0mg
Sodium	55mg
Carbohydrates	17g
Fiber	3g
Sugar	2g
Added Sugars	0g
Protein	2g

VARIATIONS ON A THEME

Home fries and hashes make an easy and inexpensive breakfast and can be crafted using almost anything. Instead of standard potatoes, try making home fries with sweet potatoes, crumbled soy bacon, and leeks. Dice leftover hard-boiled eggs and/or low-sodium cheese and add to the mix. Or shred a big variety of vegetables and make yourself a super-vegan hash.

Spicy Chickpea Tacos with Arugula

These may be the tastiest tacos ever! A thick and spicy sauce dotted with meaty garbanzos, the peppery cool of arugula, and crunchy bite of corn taco shells. Spoon extra filling over cooked brown rice if you run short of shells.

2 (15-ounce) cans low-sodium chickpeas, drained and rinsed

¼ cup tomato paste

1 (8-ounce) can tomato sauce

1 tablespoon apple cider vinegar

1 tablespoon light brown sugar or brown sugar–style erythritol

2 teaspoons chili powder

1 tablespoon Dijon mustard

1 teaspoon onion powder

½ teaspoon garlic powder

¼ teaspoon ground black pepper

⅛ teaspoon red pepper flakes

12 hard corn taco shells

3 cups baby arugula

¼ cup chopped fresh cilantro

1 In a medium saucepan, add all ingredients except taco shells, arugula, and cilantro and stir well to combine.

2 Place pan over medium heat and simmer, stirring frequently, 10 minutes. Remove from heat.

3 Fill taco shells with arugula and spoon bean mixture over top. Garnish with cilantro and serve.

CHAPTER 7

Soups and Stews

Spicy Butternut Squash and Pear Soup

SERVES 6	
Per Serving (1 cup):	
Calories	120
Fat	6g
Saturated Fat	1g
Cholesterol	0mg
Sodium	135mg
Carbohydrates	15g
Fiber	4g
Sugar	5g
Added Sugars	0g
Protein	3g

This twist on butternut squash soup is both spicy and sweet. Top with pumpkin seeds, pistachios, or any other favorite nuts or seeds. Serve some in small bowls as an appetizer for a party or meal prep for a week of healthy lunches.

3 cups frozen cubed butternut squash

2 tablespoons extra-virgin olive oil, divided

½ teaspoon kosher salt

1 small onion, peeled and sliced (approximately 1 cup)

1 medium pear, cored and cut into cubes

2¼ cups low-sodium chicken or vegetable broth

⅛ teaspoon ground black pepper

⅛ teaspoon ground cumin

⅛ teaspoon ground cayenne pepper

½ cup unsweetened vanilla almond milk

2 tablespoons roasted shelled pumpkin seeds

1 Preheat oven to 400°F. In a medium microwave-safe bowl, microwave butternut squash according to package directions, approximately 7–9 minutes. Add 1 tablespoon oil and salt and toss squash together to mix; set aside.

2 Meanwhile, heat remaining 1 tablespoon oil in a large stockpot over medium heat. Add onion and pear and sauté 3 minutes. Add broth, black pepper, cumin, and cayenne and heat through 2 minutes.

3 Add squash and heat through 2–3 minutes. Turn off heat.

4 Use an immersion blender or add mixture to a kitchen blender and purée until smooth. Once desired consistency is reached, blend in milk.

5 Pour into six medium bowls and garnish each serving with 1 teaspoon pumpkin seeds. Serve.

Spicy Cauliflower and Mushroom Soup

Soup lovers need no coaxing, but studies have shown that individuals who consume soup almost daily are more likely to have a lower BMI. Also, when soup is enjoyed at the start of a meal, it often results in fewer total calories consumed at that meal. Add this vegetable-packed soup to your rotation to warm up on cool days. If almond milk isn't your thing, you can also use cashew or soy milk.

1 tablespoon olive oil

1 medium yellow onion, peeled and chopped

4 cups riced cauliflower

8 ounces white mushrooms, thinly sliced

4 cups low-sodium chicken or vegetable broth

½ teaspoon kosher salt

¼ teaspoon ground black pepper

¼ teaspoon ground smoked paprika

½ cup unsweetened almond milk

1. In a large pot over medium-high heat, heat oil. Add onion and sauté until translucent, about 5 minutes.
2. Add cauliflower and cook 3 minutes. Add mushrooms and sauté an additional 7–8 minutes.
3. Add broth, salt, black pepper, and smoked paprika and bring to a boil; cook 5 more minutes.
4. Turn off heat, stir in almond milk, and blend in pot with an immersion blender until desired consistency is achieved. You may also transfer soup to a blender or food processor and pulse until smooth. Serve.

SERVES 6

Per Serving (1 cup):

Calories	70
Fat	2.5g
Saturated Fat	0g
Cholesterol	0mg
Sodium	180mg
Carbohydrates	7g
Fiber	2g
Sugar	3g
Added Sugars	0g
Protein	4g

TIP

This soup can be served chunky or smooth depending on which texture you prefer. Hold back a few cooked mushrooms and add them after blending if you want some chewiness.

Tuscan Pasta Fagioli

SERVES 8

Per Serving (1 cup):

Calories	230
Fat	5g
Saturated Fat	1.5g
Cholesterol	5mg
Sodium	430mg
Carbohydrates	37g
Fiber	7g
Sugar	3g
Added Sugars	0g
Protein	10g

This hearty soup brings restaurant quality into your kitchen. It's super satisfying on its own or you can add rotisserie chicken or another preferred protein source to make a complete entrée for dinner.

2 tablespoons olive oil

⅓ cup chopped onion

3 medium cloves garlic, peeled and minced

1 (8-ounce) can diced tomatoes, undrained

5 cups low-sodium vegetable broth

¼ teaspoon ground black pepper

1 teaspoon kosher salt

½ teaspoon dried oregano

¼ teaspoon red pepper flakes

2 teaspoons lemon juice

¼ cup chopped fresh parsley

2 (15-ounce) cans cannellini beans, drained and rinsed, divided

2½ cups dry whole-grain pasta shells

3 tablespoons grated Parmesan cheese

1. In a large pot over medium heat, heat oil. Add onion and garlic and cook until soft but not browned, about 5 minutes. Add tomatoes with juice, broth, black pepper, salt, oregano, red pepper flakes, lemon juice, and parsley.
2. In a food processor or blender, blend 1½ cups cannellini beans, adding small amounts of hot broth or water to make a smooth purée. Add puréed beans to broth mixture and stir. Cover and simmer 20 minutes.
3. While broth is simmering, cook pasta until al dente and drain.
4. Add remaining beans and pasta to pot and heat through 2–3 minutes. Pour into bowls and sprinkle with Parmesan before serving.

Classic Chicken Noodle Soup

No cookbook would be complete without this perennial favorite. This low-fat, lower-sodium version makes the most of meaty chicken and tender vegetables. Add more broth to increase the volume if you prefer.

2 cups shredded cooked chicken

2 medium carrots, peeled and sliced

1 medium stalk celery, sliced

1 small onion, peeled and diced

3 medium cloves garlic, peeled and minced

4 cups low-sodium chicken broth

1 teaspoon all-purpose seasoning

½ teaspoon ground sage

¼ teaspoon ground rosemary

⅛ teaspoon ground black pepper

1½ cups dry whole-grain egg noodles

1 In a large stockpot over high heat, combine all ingredients except noodles. Bring to a boil.

2 Once boiling, add noodles, reduce heat to medium-low, and simmer 10 minutes.

3 Remove from heat. Ladle soup into four medium bowls and serve immediately.

SERVES 4	
Per Serving:	
Calories	210
Fat	3g
Saturated Fat	0.5g
Cholesterol	70mg
Sodium	570mg
Carbohydrates	19g
Fiber	4g
Sugar	3g
Added Sugars	0g
Protein	26g

Chicken Soup with Jalapeño and Lime

Per Serving:

Calories	110
Fat	1.5g
Saturated Fat	0g
Cholesterol	35mg
Sodium	310mg
Carbohydrates	8g
Fiber	2g
Sugar	3g
Added Sugars	0g
Protein	14g

Set your taste buds abuzz with the zing of fresh lime! This low-sodium soup is brimming over with flavor, yet virtually fat free. For added heft, ladle soup over bowls of cooked whole-grain noodles or brown or wild rice.

2 cups shredded cooked chicken

1 medium red onion, peeled and diced

3 medium cloves garlic, peeled and minced

2 medium carrots, peeled and sliced

1 medium stalk celery, sliced

1 medium red bell pepper, seeded and diced

2 tablespoons minced jalapeño pepper

1 (15-ounce) can diced tomatoes, undrained

Juice of 2 medium limes (about ¼ cup)

8 cups low-sodium chicken broth

1 teaspoon ground cumin

½ teaspoon ground coriander

¼ teaspoon dried oregano

⅛ teaspoon ground black pepper

2 tablespoons chopped fresh cilantro

1 medium lime, cut into wedges

1 In a large stockpot over high heat, add all ingredients except cilantro and lime wedges. Bring to a boil.

2 Once boiling, reduce heat to low, cover, and simmer 15 minutes.

3 Remove from heat, ladle into medium bowls, and garnish with cilantro and lime wedges. Serve immediately.

Garden Tomato Soup

Ripe tomatoes, sweet bell pepper, and onion partner perfectly in this fresh vegetable soup. Serve with high-fiber grilled cheese sandwiches for sensational comfort food.

1 tablespoon olive oil

3 cups peeled, chopped, and seeded tomatoes

1 cup chopped onion

1 cup chopped red bell pepper

1 tablespoon minced garlic

4 cups low-sodium vegetable broth

2 tablespoons tomato paste

1 tablespoon chopped fresh basil

1 teaspoon chopped fresh oregano

½ teaspoon chopped fresh thyme

⅛ teaspoon ground black pepper

SERVES 4	
Per Serving:	
Calories	110
Fat	4.5g
Saturated Fat	0.5g
Cholesterol	0mg
Sodium	135mg
Carbohydrates	15g
Fiber	4g
Sugar	9g
Added Sugars	1g
Protein	2g

1 In a large stockpot over medium heat, heat oil. Add tomatoes, onion, bell pepper, and garlic and cook, stirring, 10 minutes.
2 Add remaining ingredients and stir to combine. Turn heat to high and bring to a boil.
3 Once boiling, reduce heat to low, cover, and simmer 10 minutes.
4 Remove from heat. Transfer mixture to a blender or food processor and purée until smooth. Serve immediately.

Easy Wonton Soup

SERVES 8

Per Serving:

Calories	160
Fat	5g
Saturated Fat	1.5g
Cholesterol	20mg
Sodium	100mg
Carbohydrates	19g
Fiber	2g
Sugar	1g
Added Sugars	0g
Protein	11g

This low-sodium soup mimics the classic wonton so much you'll be hard pressed to tell the difference. Add your choice of fresh mushrooms—from basic white button or baby bella to oyster or shiitake.

8 ounces lean ground pork

1 tablespoon minced fresh ginger

4 medium cloves garlic, peeled and minced

8 cups low-sodium chicken broth

2 cups sliced mushrooms

6 ounces dry whole-grain egg noodles

¼ teaspoon ground white pepper

4 medium scallions, chopped

1 Place a large stockpot over medium heat. Add pork, ginger, and garlic and sauté 5 minutes. Drain any excess fat and return to stovetop over medium heat.

2 Add broth and bring to a boil. Once boiling, stir in mushrooms, noodles, and white pepper. Cover and simmer 10 minutes.

3 Remove stockpot from heat. Stir in scallions and serve immediately.

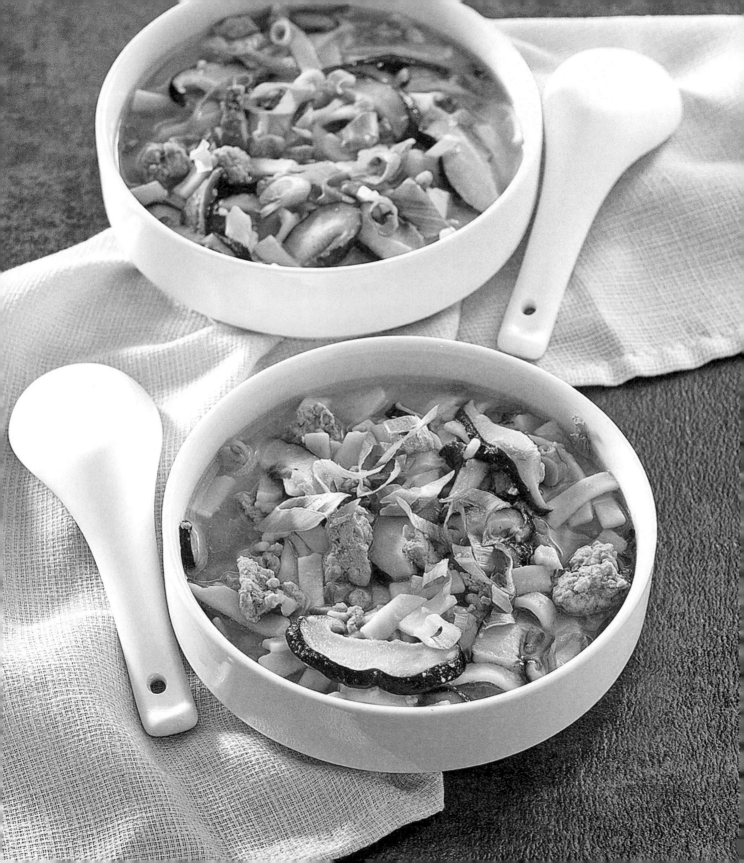

Tofu Soup

GINGER FACTS

Ginger, also called gingerroot, has been used for hundreds of years as a natural remedy for many ailments, particularly nausea. It can be eaten raw, cooked, or ground, and adds a spicy, distinctive flavor to both sweet and savory dishes. Ginger contains antioxidants and anti-inflammatory compounds believed to inhibit cancer and cardiovascular disease.

This low-sodium soup is a natural cure-all. Meaty chunks of tofu and vegetables are bathed in a soft broth with a slightly spicy kick.

8 cups low-sodium vegetable broth

3 medium carrots, peeled and diced

4 ounces mushrooms, sliced

6 medium scallions, sliced, divided

8 medium cloves garlic, peeled and minced

1 (1") piece fresh ginger, minced

¼ teaspoon ground white pepper

1 pound extra-firm tofu, drained and cut into cubes

1 In a large stockpot over high heat, add broth, carrots, mushrooms, 4 scallions, garlic, ginger, and white pepper. Bring to a boil.

2 Once boiling, add tofu. Reduce heat to low, cover, and simmer 5 minutes.

3 Remove from heat, ladle soup into medium bowls, and garnish with remaining 2 scallions. Serve immediately.

White Bean and Collard Green Soup

Beans and greens are a fabulous pairing for a nutrient-packed soup. Use any hearty greens you like such as kale or Swiss chard.

1 tablespoon olive oil

1 cup finely chopped yellow onion

4 medium cloves garlic, peeled and minced

½ cup dry white wine

¼ teaspoon ground black pepper

¼ teaspoon kosher salt

4 cups thinly shredded collard greens

¾ teaspoon dried thyme

4 cups low-sodium chicken broth

1 (15-ounce) can low-sodium cannellini or great northern beans, drained and rinsed

1 teaspoon red wine vinegar

SERVES 4	
Per Serving:	
Calories	180
Fat	4g
Saturated Fat	1g
Cholesterol	0mg
Sodium	270mg
Carbohydrates	22g
Fiber	6g
Sugar	3g
Added Sugars	0g
Protein	9g

1 In a large pot over medium heat, heat oil. Add onion and garlic and sauté 5 minutes or until onion is tender.

2 Add wine, black pepper, and salt and reduce heat to a simmer for 5 minutes or until wine mostly evaporates.

3 Add greens, thyme, and broth. Cover and cook 8 minutes or until greens are tender.

4 Add beans and vinegar and heat through, about 5 minutes. Serve.

Vegetable and Bean Chili Soup

SERVES 8

Per Serving (1 cup):

Calories	170
Fat	3.5g
Saturated Fat	1g
Cholesterol	0mg
Sodium	150mg
Carbohydrates	29g
Fiber	8g
Sugar	10g
Added Sugars	2g
Protein	8g

An easy meal for Meatless Monday or a vegetarian crowd, this vegetarian chili is warm and nourishing. Freeze extras to keep on hand when your grocery stash runs low. You can include the jalapeño seeds if you like the chili extra hot. Suggested toppings are reduced-fat shredded Mexican or Cheddar cheese and avocado.

4 teaspoons olive oil

2 cups chopped onions

½ cup chopped green bell pepper

3 medium cloves garlic, peeled and chopped

1 small jalapeño pepper, seeded and finely chopped

1 tablespoon chili powder

1 teaspoon ground cumin

2 (28-ounce) cans low-sodium chopped tomatoes, undrained

1 medium zucchini, diced

2 (15-ounce) cans low-sodium red kidney beans, drained and rinsed

1 tablespoon chopped semisweet chocolate

3 tablespoons chopped fresh cilantro

1 Heat a large pot over medium-high heat. Add oil, onions, bell pepper, garlic, and jalapeño and sauté until vegetables are softened, about 5 minutes. Add chili powder and cumin and sauté 1 minute, stirring frequently to mix well.

2 Add tomatoes with juice and zucchini and bring to a boil. Reduce heat to low and simmer, partially covered, 10 minutes, stirring occasionally.

3 Stir in beans and chocolate and simmer, stirring occasionally, an additional 10 minutes or until beans are heated through and chocolate is melted.

4 Stir in cilantro and serve.

Winter White Turkey Chili

Cozy comfort food for a crowd! Spruce up this easy chili by serving it with sliced avocado, reduced-fat shredded Cheddar cheese, and fresh cilantro. Pair with a piece of Perfect Corn Bread (see Chapter 10) for a fun family dinner.

2 teaspoons olive oil

1⅓ pounds 93% lean ground turkey

1 cup chopped onion

1 (4-ounce) can diced green chilies, drained

¾ teaspoon dried oregano

¾ teaspoon ground cumin

¼ teaspoon ground cayenne pepper

2 (15-ounce) cans low-sodium great northern beans, drained and rinsed

3 cups low-sodium chicken broth

1½ tablespoons apple cider vinegar

1 In a large pot over medium-high heat, heat oil. Place turkey on one side of the pot and onions on the other. Cook turkey undisturbed for 4 minutes while stirring onions a few times. Break up turkey to combine with onions and cook until turkey is no longer pink, about 3 minutes.

2 Add chilies, oregano, cumin, and cayenne and stir occasionally for 2 minutes.

3 Add beans and broth and bring to a simmer. Cook an additional 15 minutes to reduce liquid, stirring occasionally.

4 Add vinegar and cook an additional 3 minutes. Serve.

SERVES 6

Per Serving (1 cup):

Calories	270
Fat	9g
Saturated Fat	1.5g
Cholesterol	45mg
Sodium	330mg
Carbohydrates	24g
Fiber	5g
Sugar	3g
Added Sugars	0g
Protein	28g

VARIATIONS

The spiciness of this recipe can be easily adjusted. Some may prefer additional cayenne or hot sauce, which will not significantly alter the nutritional information. You could also add some reduced-fat shredded Cheddar cheese or light sour cream for variety.

Manhattan-Style Seafood Stew

This easy, healthy, and delicious restaurant-quality meal will be on repeat in your house. It's even better the next day after the flavors have time to meld. Switch up the seafood depending on what you have in the house or what's on sale at the supermarket.

1½ teaspoons olive oil

1 large onion, peeled and diced

4 medium cloves garlic, peeled and minced

2 (15-ounce) cans diced tomatoes, undrained

2 cups low-sodium chicken broth

2 medium carrots, peeled and thinly sliced

8 ounces white-fleshed fish such as tilapia, cut into 1" chunks

1 medium jalapeño pepper, seeded and minced

1 large bay leaf

8 ounces small shrimp, shelled

⅓ cup chopped fresh parsley

½ teaspoon orange zest

½ teaspoon ground black pepper

¼ cup grated Parmesan cheese

1 In a large stockpot or Dutch oven over medium heat, heat oil. Add onion and garlic and cook, stirring, 3 minutes.

2 Add tomatoes with juice, broth, carrots, fish, jalapeños, and bay leaf and stir to combine.

3 Cover stockpot and cook, stirring occasionally, 15 minutes.

4 Add shrimp, parsley, orange zest, and black pepper and stir well. Simmer until shrimp are pink, about 5 minutes, then remove from heat.

5 Carefully remove bay leaf and serve immediately. Top each serving with 1 tablespoon Parmesan.

Quick Minestrone Soup

This nourishing favorite is made almost entirely from pantry items for a quick meal when your groceries are running low. Substitute whatever vegetables you have on hand for a flavor twist.

2 cups diced zucchini

½ cup dry whole-wheat elbow pasta

⅛ teaspoon ground black pepper

2 medium cloves garlic, peeled and minced

4 cups low-sodium chicken broth

1 (14.5-ounce) can Italian style diced tomatoes, undrained

1 (16-ounce) can low-sodium red kidney beans, drained and rinsed

1 (10-ounce) bag frozen peas and carrots, defrosted

½ cup grated Parmesan cheese

1 In a large pot over high heat, combine all ingredients except Parmesan. Bring to a boil.

2 Once boiling, cover and reduce heat to medium-low; simmer 10 minutes, stirring occasionally until pasta is done.

3 Transfer to medium bowls and serve with 1 tablespoon Parmesan sprinkled over each serving.

SERVES 8	
Per Serving:	
Calories	140
Fat	3g
Saturated Fat	1.5g
Cholesterol	5mg
Sodium	320mg
Carbohydrates	20g
Fiber	4g
Sugar	5g
Added Sugars	1g
Protein	9g

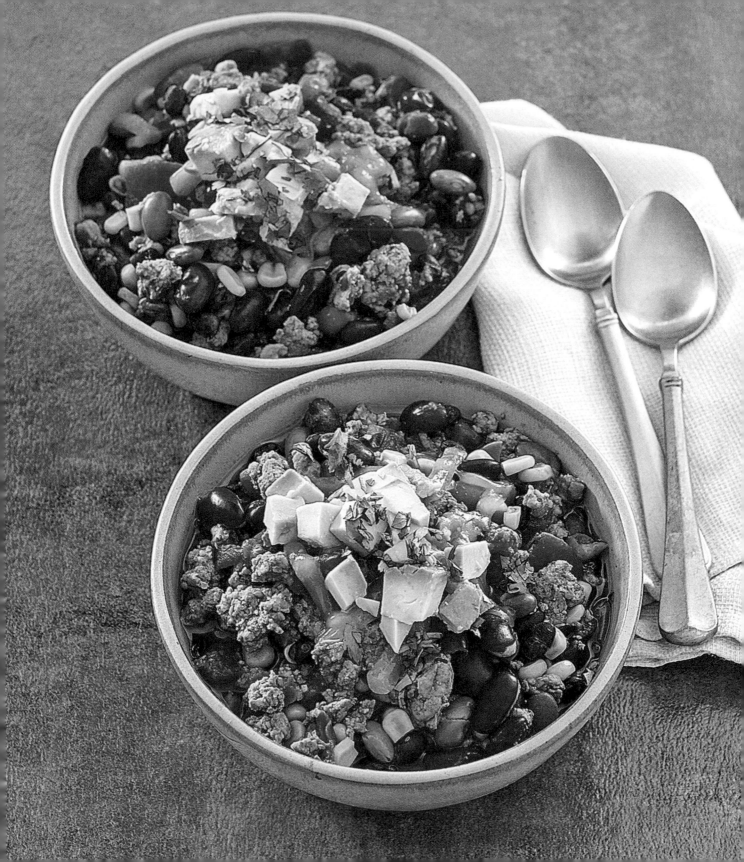

Quick Turkey Taco Soup

Super easy with no chopping necessary, this satisfying soup can be made with any variety of beans you have in the pantry. Serve this soup with reduced-fat Cheddar cheese, chopped avocado, and cilantro for a hearty lunch or dinner.

1 tablespoon olive oil

1⅓ pounds package lean ground turkey

2 (28-ounce) cans crushed tomatoes, undrained

1 (14-ounce) can low-sodium black beans, drained and rinsed

1 (14-ounce) can low-sodium pinto beans, drained and rinsed

1 (14-ounce) can low-sodium kidney beans, drained and rinsed

1 (14-ounce) can corn kernels, drained and rinsed

2 tablespoons taco seasoning, less sodium

1 In a large Dutch oven or stockpot over medium-high heat, heat oil 30 seconds. Add turkey and cook 8 minutes or until no longer pink.

2 Add tomatoes, beans, corn, and taco seasoning and stir to combine. Cook 20 minutes, stirring occasionally. Serve.

SERVES 12	
Per Serving (1 cup):	
Calories	230
Fat	6g
Saturated Fat	1g
Cholesterol	20mg
Sodium	440mg
Carbohydrates	32g
Fiber	8g
Sugar	9g
Added Sugars	0g
Protein	18g

Low-Cal Garden Soup

Six different vegetables combine with garlic and herbs to create a tasty soup that will fill you up with only a few calories. Store leftovers in an airtight container in the refrigerator up to 3 days.

1 teaspoon olive oil

¾ cup chopped white onion

1½ cups chopped celery

1½ cups chopped carrots

1½ cups chopped zucchini

1½ cups cut green beans

½ teaspoon garlic powder

1 teaspoon dried oregano

4 cups low-sodium chicken broth

1 (14-ounce) can stewed tomatoes, undrained

¼ cup chopped fresh basil

1 In a large pot over medium heat, heat oil 30 seconds. Add onion, celery, and carrots and sauté until crisp-tender, about 10 minutes.

2 Add zucchini, green beans, garlic powder, oregano, broth, and tomatoes with juice and bring to a light boil.

3 Reduce heat to low and simmer until vegetables are tender, about 10 minutes. Garnish with basil before serving.

CHAPTER 8

Pasta, Rice, and Grains

Pesto Shrimp and Vegetables over Linguine

A jar of pesto is a kitchen staple that add tons of flavor to a dish in a flash. A tablespoon goes a long way, saves time on busy evenings, and brings together most protein and vegetables into a cohesive dish.

8 ounces dry whole-wheat or fiber-enriched linguine

1 tablespoon olive oil

2 teaspoons finely chopped garlic, divided

10 ounces white mushrooms, sliced

2 cups fresh spinach

1 pound shrimp, shelled and deveined

1 cup halved grape tomatoes

¼ cup jarred pesto

4 teaspoons grated Parmesan cheese

1 In a medium pot, bring water to a boil and cook linguine according to package directions. Drain and set aside.

2 Heat a large sauté pan over medium to medium-high heat and add oil. Add 1 teaspoon garlic and cook approximately 30 seconds. Add mushrooms and sauté 3–5 minutes. Add spinach and cook until wilted, about 2–3 minutes.

3 Transfer vegetables from pan to a medium bowl using a slotted spoon, draining as you go. Pour out extra liquid from pan and add shrimp and remaining 1 teaspoon garlic. Sauté until shrimp is cooked through and no longer pink, approximately 4 minutes. If liquid remains in pan, drain it.

4 Return vegetables to pan and add tomatoes (it's okay if there's some liquid from spinach and mushrooms).

5 Add cooked pasta and pesto to pan. Gently combine and heat through for 3–4 minutes. Transfer to medium bowls, sprinkle each with 1 teaspoon Parmesan, and serve.

Fresh Tomato and Clam Sauce with Whole-Grain Linguine

Fresh clams are so simple to prepare yet they present like a fancy restaurant-style treat. Have a little extra parsley or basil ready to garnish this dish for some added flair.

3 dozen littleneck clams

2 tablespoons olive oil

5 medium cloves garlic, peeled and chopped

½ cup chopped red bell pepper

4 cups peeled and chopped tomatoes

3 tablespoons chopped fresh parsley

1 tablespoon chopped fresh basil

¼ teaspoon salt

¼ teaspoon red pepper flakes

½ teaspoon dried oregano

½ cup dry white wine

8 ounces whole-grain linguine

1. Before preparing this dish (preferably several hours or more), place clams in bowl of cold water with handful of cornmeal added; keep refrigerated. (This will help purge clams of any sand or other debris.) When ready to cook, rinse and scrub clams.

2. In a large deep skillet over medium-high heat, heat oil, garlic, and bell pepper. Add tomatoes, parsley, basil, salt, red pepper flakes, and oregano. Bring to a boil, then reduce heat to low and simmer 15–20 minutes.

3. Stir in wine and add clams on top of mixture. Cover and steam until clams open, usually 3–5 minutes. Discard any clams that do not open; they are not suitable for eating.

4. Meanwhile, in a large pot, boil water and cook linguine to al dente.

5. Serve by placing tomato sauce and clams over pasta.

SERVES 4

Per Serving:	
Calories	400
Fat	10g
Saturated Fat	1.5g
Cholesterol	25mg
Sodium	650mg
Carbohydrates	55g
Fiber	8g
Sugar	7g
Added Sugars	0g
Protein	22g

NO FRESH CLAMS? USE CANNED.

This recipe works well with canned clams if you are unable to get fresh. Canned clams are high in sodium, which will need to be taken into consideration. If you are using canned clams, you will need 1 (8-ounce) can minced clams.

Balsamic Farro with Peppers, Walnuts, and Goat Cheese

This whole-grain salad is a fantastic summer side dish to serve with grilled chicken, fish, or steak. Add it to salad greens to stretch a vegetarian meal or double the portion for a portable lunch on the go.

SERVES 4	
Per Serving:	
Calories	250
Fat	10g
Saturated Fat	2g
Cholesterol	5mg
Sodium	210mg
Carbohydrates	35g
Fiber	4g
Sugar	4g
Added Sugars	1g
Protein	9g

1 ounce walnuts, chopped

2 cups cooked farro

½ cup jarred roasted red peppers, drained and chopped

2 medium scallions, chopped

2 tablespoons crumbled goat cheese

1 tablespoon extra-virgin olive oil

2 tablespoons balsamic vinegar

1 tablespoon plain nonfat Greek yogurt

¾ teaspoon honey

1 Preheat oven or toaster oven to 350°F.

2 Toast walnuts on a small baking sheet approximately 3 minutes, taking care not to burn them.

3 In a medium bowl, add farro, walnuts, red peppers, scallions, and goat cheese and gently combine.

4 In a small bowl, add oil, vinegar, yogurt, and honey and whisk until blended.

5 Pour dressing over salad and gently mix to combine. Serve.

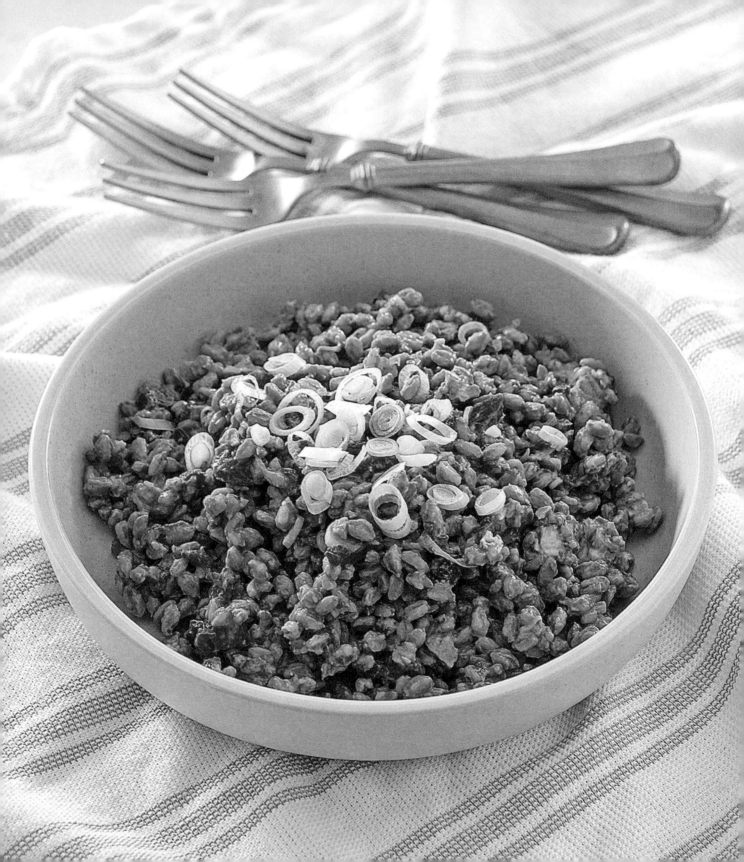

Herbed Quinoa with Sun-Dried Tomatoes

SERVES 4	
Per Serving:	
Calories	210
Fat	5g
Saturated Fat	0g
Cholesterol	0mg
Sodium	45mg
Carbohydrates	34g
Fiber	4g
Sugar	3g
Added Sugars	0g
Protein	7g

Some people shy away from quinoa because it seems exotic or hard to cook, but in reality, quinoa takes no longer to cook than rice or pasta, usually about 15 minutes. You can tell it is cooked when the grains have turned from white to transparent and the spiral-like germ has separated from the seed.

½ tablespoon olive oil

¼ cup chopped onion

1 medium clove garlic, peeled and minced

1 cup quinoa

2 cups low-sodium chicken broth

½ cup sliced mushrooms

6 medium sun-dried tomatoes, cut into ¼" pieces

1 teaspoon dried Italian seasoning

1 In a medium saucepan over medium heat, heat oil. Add onion and garlic and sauté 5 minutes.

2 Rinse quinoa in a fine-mesh strainer or coffee filter. Add quinoa and broth to pan and bring to a boil 2 minutes. Add mushrooms, sun-dried tomatoes, and Italian seasoning.

3 Reduce heat and cover. Cook 15 minutes, or until all liquid is absorbed. Serve.

Tomatoes Stuffed with Quinoa Salad

Tomatoes are fabulous vessels to stuff with any kind of grain salad for a plant-focused meal. These are visually impressive for a lunch party; make them during the summer when tomatoes are in season with beautiful color and robust flavor.

½ cup quinoa

1 cup water

6 large tomatoes (about 3 pounds)

1½ cups peeled and finely diced cucumber

⅓ cup chopped fresh parsley

¼ cup chopped fresh mint

½ cup finely chopped red onion

3 tablespoons crumbled feta cheese

2 tablespoons lemon juice

3 tablespoons olive oil

¼ teaspoon kosher salt

SERVES 6	
Per Serving:	
Calories	170
Fat	9g
Saturated Fat	2g
Cholesterol	5mg
Sodium	105mg
Carbohydrates	20g
Fiber	4g
Sugar	6g
Added Sugars	0g
Protein	4g

1 Rinse quinoa in a fine-mesh strainer or coffee filter. Place quinoa and water in a small saucepan over high heat and bring to a boil. Reduce heat, cover, and cook until all water is absorbed, about 15 minutes. Let cool at least 15 minutes.

2 Remove caps of tomatoes and hollow out, leaving shell about ½" thick.

3 In a medium bowl, combine cooked quinoa, cucumber, parsley, mint, onion, and feta.

4 In a small bowl, mix lemon juice, oil, and salt. Pour over quinoa and vegetables.

5 Stuff tomatoes with mixture and serve.

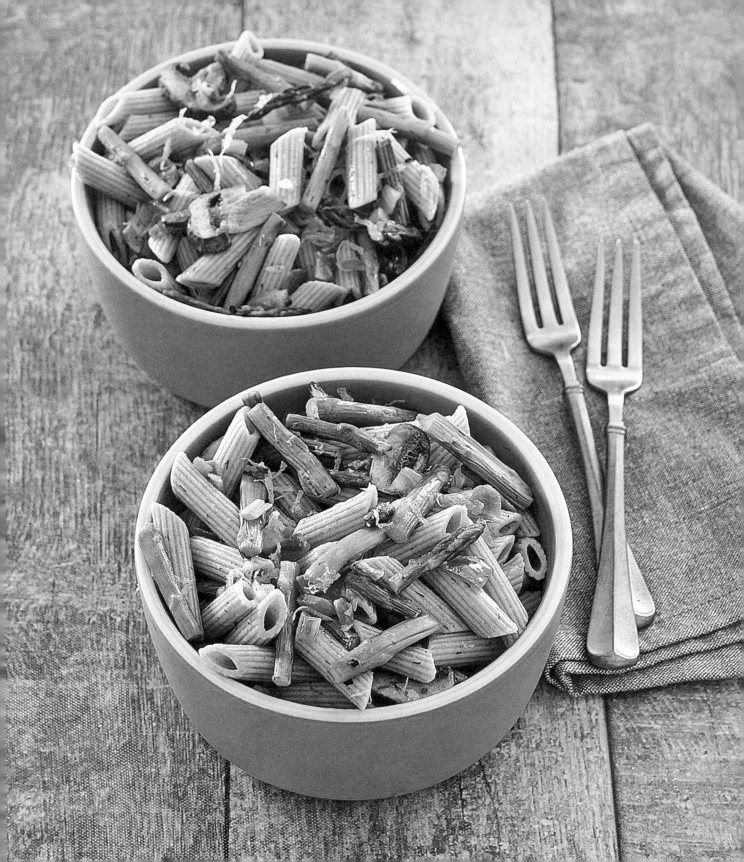

Whole-Grain Penne with Lemony Roasted Asparagus

In this recipe, oven roasting draws out depth in the vegetables, which is punctuated by a citrus burst. Pump up the protein with no fuss by adding leftover rotisserie chicken or canned tuna or salmon for a complete, balanced meal.

12 ounces asparagus, trimmed and cut into 2" pieces

8 ounces mushrooms, thickly sliced

½ medium red onion, peeled and diced

2 teaspoons olive oil

3 tablespoons lemon juice, divided

¼ teaspoon ground black pepper, divided

8 ounces dry whole-grain penne

1 tablespoon lemon zest

¼ teaspoon kosher salt

½ teaspoon dried dill

SERVES 4	
Per Serving:	
Calories	260
Fat	4g
Saturated Fat	0.5g
Cholesterol	0mg
Sodium	85mg
Carbohydrates	50g
Fiber	8g
Sugar	5g
Added Sugars	0g
Protein	12g

1 Preheat oven to 450°F. Line a large baking sheet with aluminum foil and set aside.

2 In a medium bowl, place asparagus, mushrooms, and onion. Add oil, 2 tablespoons lemon juice, and ⅛ teaspoon black pepper and toss to coat.

3 Spread mixture onto prepared baking sheet. Place on middle rack in oven and bake 20 minutes.

4 In a large pot, bring water to a boil and cook penne according to package directions, omitting salt. Drain.

5 Once vegetables are roasted, add to cooked pasta, along with all cooking juices. Add remaining 1 tablespoon lemon juice and zest and toss to coat. Season with salt, dill, and remaining ⅛ teaspoon black pepper. Serve immediately.

Sweet Sorghum Salad with Apples, Pine Nuts, and Raisins

Per Serving (rounded ½ cup):

Calories	220
Fat	9g
Saturated Fat	1.5g
Cholesterol	0mg
Sodium	50mg
Carbohydrates	33g
Fiber	4g
Sugar	9g
Added Sugars	2g
Protein	4g

TOASTING PINE NUTS

To toast your pine nuts: Place them in a toaster oven (or regular oven) at 350°F on aluminum foil and toast about 3 minutes, watching to make sure they do not burn. As an alternative, you can toast them in a dry skillet over medium-high heat until they are slightly browned and fragrant.

Switch up your holiday side dishes with this satisfying grain salad that pairs well with any meal from summer barbecues to Thanksgiving tables. Cook a larger batch of sorghum in advance; it will hold its texture and won't get soggy in the refrigerator so you can use it all week.

3 cups packed cooked whole-grain sorghum

2 tablespoons chopped fresh parsley

1 teaspoon chopped dried rosemary

⅛ teaspoon dried thyme

½ medium apple, cored and chopped into small pieces

¼ cup packed raisins

¼ cup pine nuts, toasted

2 tablespoons apple cider vinegar

1 tablespoon pure maple syrup (or sugar-free)

¼ teaspoon kosher salt

¼ teaspoon ground black pepper

2 tablespoons extra-virgin olive oil

1 Place sorghum in a medium bowl. Add parsley, rosemary, thyme, apple, raisins, and pine nuts and toss.

2 In a small bowl, add vinegar, syrup, salt, and black pepper. Whisk in oil until well combined.

3 Pour dressing over sorghum mixture and gently mix to evenly coat. Give salad time to cool and let flavor develop before serving. It's wonderful the next day!

Pasta and Sardines with Lemon Pesto

Canned seafood is a treasure when trying to reach your goal of 8–12 ounces of seafood per week based on the US Dietary Guidelines. Sardines complement the lemon pesto beautifully, and nothing is easier than opening a can.

2 medium cloves garlic, peeled

2 cups tightly packed fresh basil leaves

¼ cup walnuts, toasted

1 tablespoon lemon juice

1 tablespoon water

½ teaspoon kosher salt

¼ teaspoon ground black pepper, plus more for serving

1 tablespoon plus 2 teaspoons olive oil

4 tablespoons grated Parmesan cheese, divided

8 ounces dry whole-grain, fiber-enriched, or bean-based pasta

2 (3-ounce) cans water-packed sardines, drained

1 Place garlic into a food processor and pulse until finely chopped. Add basil, walnuts, lemon juice, water, salt, and black pepper and process until just puréed.

2 Add oil and 3 tablespoons Parmesan. Pulse until pesto is smooth, scraping down sides of bowl as needed. Set aside.

3 In a medium pot, bring water to a boil and cook pasta according to package directions. Meanwhile, use a fork to flake sardines into a small bowl.

4 When pasta is cooked, drain and return to pot. Toss pesto and sardines with pasta and transfer to medium serving bowls. Sprinkle remaining 1 tablespoon Parmesan and some black pepper on top of each serving.

SERVES 4

Per Serving:

Calories	400
Fat	17g
Saturated Fat	4g
Cholesterol	65mg
Sodium	390mg
Carbohydrates	44g
Fiber	6g
Sugar	2g
Added Sugars	0g
Protein	22g

SARDINE NUTRITION

Sardines today are not the ones you remember from decades ago. They are meaty and so nutritious, and an excellent source of seven vitamins and minerals, including calcium and vitamin D as well as heart-healthy omega-3 fats. They are also very low in mercury.

Wild Rice Salad with Black Beans, Mango, and Lime

SERVES 6	
Per Serving:	
Calories	190
Fat	1g
Saturated Fat	0g
Cholesterol	0mg
Sodium	110mg
Carbohydrates	39g
Fiber	7g
Sugar	10g
Added Sugars	0g
Protein	8g

Delicious warm or cold, this salad showcases simple, fresh flavors the best way possible: naked! Use whichever rice you prefer— brown, basmati, jasmine, even black rice—all work well though wild and black/forbidden rice provide the richest nutrient content.

3 cups cooked wild rice

1 (15-ounce) can low-sodium black beans, drained and rinsed

1 medium ripe mango, peeled, pitted, and diced

1 medium red bell pepper, seeded and diced

2 medium scallions, sliced

2 medium cloves garlic, peeled and minced

Juice of 2 medium limes

¼ cup chopped fresh cilantro

⅛ teaspoon kosher salt

⅛ teaspoon ground black pepper

1 In a medium mixing bowl, add all ingredients and stir well to combine.

2 Serve immediately or cover and refrigerate until ready to serve.

Tuna Pasta Salad with Broccoli and Sun-Dried Tomatoes

Bold flavors combine flawlessly in this healthy pasta salad. With whole-grain, low-fat protein, vitamins, and nutrients, it's a one-dish meal that's wonderful served warm or cold.

½ cup chopped sun-dried tomatoes (not in oil)

1 cup boiling water

12 ounces dry whole-grain penne

1 tablespoon olive oil

1 medium head broccoli, cut into small florets

2 medium scallions, finely diced

2 (5-ounce) cans water-packed no-salt-added solid white tuna, drained

2 tablespoons balsamic vinegar

½ teaspoon kosher salt

½ teaspoon ground black pepper

SERVES 8	
Per Serving:	
Calories	250
Fat	6g
Saturated Fat	1g
Cholesterol	20mg
Sodium	160mg
Carbohydrates	36g
Fiber	5g
Sugar	4g
Added Sugars	0g
Protein	17g

1. Place sun-dried tomatoes in a small bowl, add boiling water, and let soak 10 minutes. Drain and reserve 2 tablespoons of soaking liquid.

2. In a large pot, bring water to a boil and cook penne according to package directions, omitting salt. Drain and set aside.

3. In a large sauté pan over medium heat, heat oil. Add broccoli and sauté 5 minutes. Remove pan from heat.

4. Add sun-dried tomatoes, reserved soaking liquid, penne, scallions, tuna, vinegar, salt, and black pepper to pan and stir well to combine.

5. Serve immediately or cover and refrigerate until ready to serve.

Spicy Thai Peanut Noodles

Whip up these spicy noodles to make a satisfying and delicious meatless meal. For more protein and fiber, try bean-based pasta. When enjoying leftovers, add more broth to moisten when reheating.

1 pound dry whole-grain angel hair or thin spaghetti pasta

3 teaspoons sesame oil, divided

1 small red onion, peeled and diced

4 medium cloves garlic, peeled and minced

1 tablespoon minced fresh ginger

1 medium red bell pepper, seeded and diced

½ cup low-sodium vegetable broth

2 tablespoons natural peanut butter, no added sugar

2 tablespoons lime juice

½ teaspoon red pepper flakes

3 medium scallions, chopped

¼ cup chopped peanuts

1 In a large pot, bring water to a boil and cook pasta according to package directions, omitting salt. Drain. Add 1 teaspoon oil to cooked pasta and toss well to coat. Set aside.

2 In a medium sauté pan over medium heat, heat remaining 2 teaspoons oil. Add onion, garlic, and ginger and sauté 2 minutes.

3 Add bell pepper and sauté 3 minutes. Remove pan from heat.

4 Stir in broth, peanut butter, lime juice, red pepper flakes, scallions, and peanuts.

5 Add pasta and toss well to coat. Serve immediately.

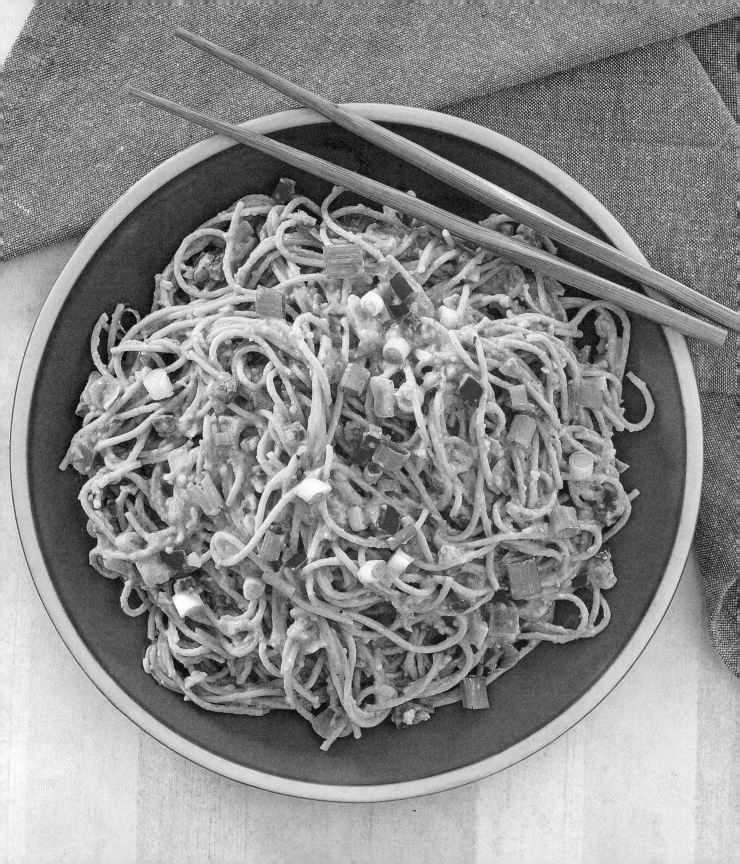

Sesame Shrimp and Asparagus

SERVES 4

Per Serving:

Calories	280
Fat	6g
Saturated Fat	1g
Cholesterol	230mg
Sodium	340mg
Carbohydrates	25g
Fiber	4g
Sugar	2g
Added Sugars	0g
Protein	34g

Seafood, vegetables, and pasta make a flavorful partnership in this dish. For a lower-carb meal, try substituting bean-based pasta, shirataki noodles, or hearts of palm "pasta."

2 teaspoons olive oil

2 medium cloves garlic, peeled and chopped

1 tablespoon grated fresh ginger

1¼ pounds medium shrimp, shelled and deveined

2 tablespoons dry white wine

8 ounces asparagus, cut diagonally into 1" pieces

2 cups cooked whole-grain pasta

½ teaspoon sesame seeds

¼ cup thinly sliced scallions

1 teaspoon sesame oil

¼ teaspoon red pepper flakes

⅛ teaspoon ground black pepper

1 Heat olive oil in a large nonstick skillet or wok over high heat. Add garlic, ginger, and shrimp and stir-fry until shrimp begins to turn pink, about 2 minutes.

2 Add wine and asparagus and stir-fry an additional 3–5 minutes.

3 Add pasta, sesame seeds, scallions, sesame oil, and red pepper flakes. Toss lightly to combine, add black pepper, and serve.

Whole-Wheat Couscous Salad with Citrus and Cilantro

This whole-grain salad strikes the perfect balance between light and filling. Its refreshing taste can be enjoyed year-round, but is best in summer with produce picked fresh from the garden.

1½ cups water

1 cup whole-wheat couscous

1 medium cucumber

1 pint grape or cherry tomatoes, halved

1 medium jalapeño pepper, seeded and minced

2 medium shallots, peeled and minced

2 medium scallions, sliced

2 medium cloves garlic, peeled and minced

2 tablespoons lemon juice

2 tablespoons lime juice

1 teaspoon olive oil

¼ cup chopped fresh cilantro

⅛ teaspoon ground black pepper

SERVES 4	
Per Serving:	
Calories	220
Fat	2g
Saturated Fat	0g
Cholesterol	0mg
Sodium	25mg
Carbohydrates	47g
Fiber	8g
Sugar	7g
Added Sugars	0g
Protein	9g

1 In a medium saucepan, bring water to a boil over high heat. Once boiling, stir in couscous. Reduce heat to medium-low, cover, and simmer 2 minutes.

2 Remove pot from heat, remove lid, and fluff couscous with a fork. Set aside to cool 5 minutes.

3 Peel cucumber and slice in half lengthwise. Use a spoon to gently scrape out and discard the seeds, then dice and place into a large mixing bowl.

4 Add remaining ingredients except black pepper to bowl along with cooked couscous. Toss well to coat.

5 Season with black pepper. Serve immediately or cover and refrigerate until ready to serve.

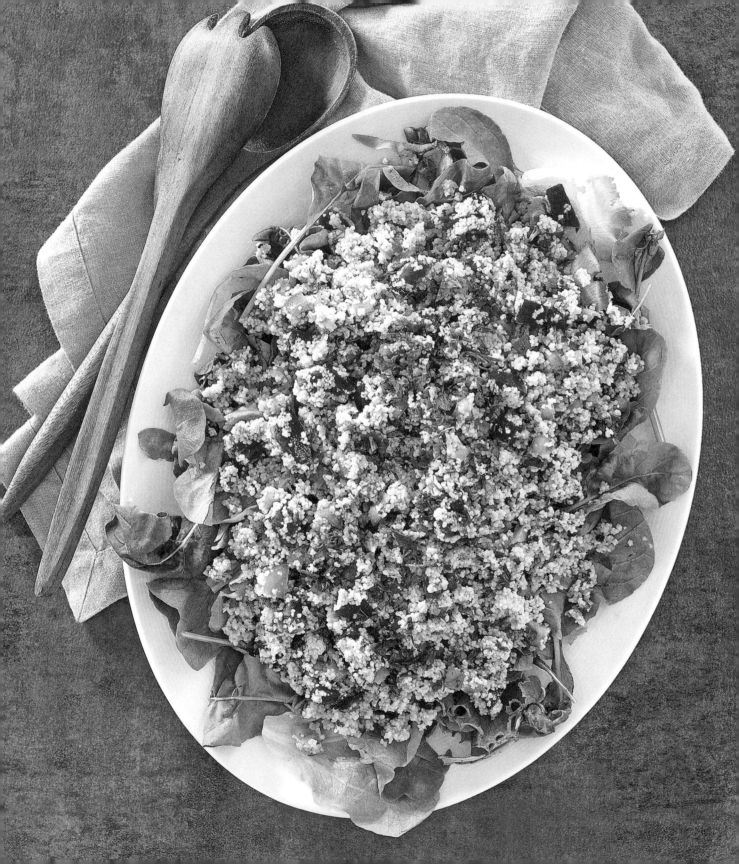

Tabouleh Salad

This refreshing salad is a wonderful way to start any meal. Serve it over a bed of lettuce for visual appeal. Or for a party, pair fresh vegetables with tabouleh and a bowl of homemade hummus.

⅔ cup whole-wheat couscous

1 cup boiling water

1 small ripe tomato, diced

1 small green bell pepper, seeded and diced

1 medium shallot, peeled and finely diced

⅓ cup chopped fresh parsley

1 medium clove garlic, peeled and minced

3 tablespoons lemon juice

1 tablespoon olive oil

¼ teaspoon kosher salt

½ teaspoon ground black pepper

1 Place couscous in a small bowl. Stir in boiling water, cover, and set aside 5 minutes.

2 In a medium salad bowl, add tomato, bell pepper, shallot, and parsley.

3 In a small mixing bowl, add garlic, lemon juice, oil, salt, and black pepper and whisk well to combine.

4 Add cooked couscous to salad bowl. Pour dressing over top and stir well to combine. Serve immediately or cover and refrigerate until ready to serve.

SERVES 4

Per Serving:

Calories	160
Fat	4g
Saturated Fat	0.5g
Cholesterol	0mg
Sodium	80mg
Carbohydrates	27g
Fiber	5g
Sugar	4g
Added Sugars	0g
Protein	5g

PARSLEY FACTS

Parsley is an easy-to-grow herb that comes in two varieties: flat-leaf and curly. Too often it's dismissed as a bland plate garnish, but parsley has amazing, distinctive flavor when eaten raw. Use it to add refreshing taste and color to salads, dressings, and pastas. Parsley contains high levels of vitamins A, C, and K as well as antioxidants, and may help prevent cardiovascular disease.

Quick and Light Baked Eggplant Parmesan Pasta

From its crisp eggplant croutons and fresh basil taste to its quick preparation time, this guilt-free version of the perennial favorite makes a protein- and fiber-packed meatless meal.

SERVES 4	
Per Serving:	
Calories	360
Fat	10g
Saturated Fat	2.5g
Cholesterol	10mg
Sodium	280mg
Carbohydrates	55g
Fiber	10g
Sugar	12g
Added Sugars	3g
Protein	17g

8 ounces dry chickpea pasta

1 medium eggplant, cut into 1" cubes

⅓ cup Homemade High-Fiber Bread Crumbs (see Chapter 9)

1 teaspoon dried Italian seasoning

¼ teaspoon kosher salt

¼ teaspoon ground black pepper

1 tablespoon olive oil

2 cups low-sodium marinara sauce

¼ cup grated Parmesan cheese

2 tablespoons chopped fresh basil

1 Preheat oven to 425°F. Spray a medium rimmed baking sheet with nonstick cooking spray and set aside.

2 In a large pot, bring water to a boil and cook pasta according to package directions, omitting salt.

3 In a large mixing bowl, add eggplant, Homemade High-Fiber Bread Crumbs, Italian seasoning, salt, black pepper, and oil. Toss well to coat.

4 Arrange eggplant mixture in a single layer on prepared baking sheet. Spay top with nonstick cooking spray. Place on middle rack in oven and bake 15 minutes.

5 Remove pan from oven. Top pasta with baked eggplant and cover with sauce, Parmesan, and basil. Serve immediately.

CHAPTER 9
Salads, Dressings, and Salsas

Beet, Orange, and Goat Cheese Salad with Citrus Vinaigrette

SERVES 2

Per Serving:

Calories	210
Fat	11g
Saturated Fat	2.5g
Cholesterol	10mg
Sodium	240mg
Carbohydrates	25g
Fiber	5g
Sugar	18g
Added Sugars	2g
Protein	5g

HOW TO ROAST BEETS

To roast fresh beets, first scrub them well, then place in foil and seal foil like a packet. Place in 400°F oven for approximately 1 hour or until tender. Wait until cool enough to handle and peel. Wear gloves to keep your hands from turning purple.

This salad feels like something you would find at a fancy spa. It's a light and fresh starter as is, or you can add some extra protein for a complete meal. To learn how to roast your own beets, see the sidebar.

2 cups mixed salad greens

2 medium packaged roasted beets, sliced into medallions

1 large orange, peeled, outer membrane removed, sliced into medallions

2 tablespoons crumbled goat cheese

2 tablespoons chopped toasted walnuts

3 tablespoons Citrus Vinaigrette (see recipe in this chapter)

1 Spread greens on a large dinner plate. Alternate beet and orange slices around the perimeter of plate. If beet slices remain, chop them into small pieces and sprinkle on the center of the greens.

2 Scatter on goat cheese and walnuts and drizzle with dressing. Serve.

Citrus Vinaigrette

Using juice in salad dressing allows for great flavor with much less oil. A little goes a long way and the sugar is minimal.

2 tablespoons extra-virgin olive oil

2 tablespoons red wine vinegar

¼ cup orange juice

2 teaspoons honey

¼ teaspoon kosher salt

2 medium cloves garlic, peeled and finely chopped

In a small container, whisk ingredients together. Serve. Cover and refrigerate leftovers for several days.

SERVES 4	
Per Serving (2 tablespoons):	
Calories	80
Fat	7g
Saturated Fat	1.5g
Cholesterol	0mg
Sodium	70mg
Carbohydrates	5g
Fiber	0g
Sugar	4g
Added Sugars	3g
Protein	0g

Bleu Cheese Dressing

Typically made with full-fat mayonnaise and sour cream, traditional bleu cheese dressing is very high in saturated fat and calories. Subbing in Greek yogurt and cottage cheese maintains creaminess with only a little mayonnaise needed.

2 tablespoons plain nonfat Greek yogurt

1 tablespoon low-fat cottage cheese

1 tablespoon light mayonnaise

½ teaspoon lemon juice

½ teaspoon honey

1 tablespoon plus 2 teaspoons crumbled bleu cheese

In a blender or food processor, place yogurt, cottage cheese, mayonnaise, lemon juice, and honey and process until smooth. Fold in bleu cheese. Serve.

SERVES 6	
Per Serving (1 tablespoon):	
Calories	20
Fat	1.5g
Saturated Fat	0.5g
Cholesterol	5mg
Sodium	55mg
Carbohydrates	1g
Fiber	0g
Sugar	1g
Added Sugars	0g
Protein	1g

Spinach Salad with Warm Citrus Vinaigrette

There's something very cozy about a warm salad dressing on a cool day. For a heartier meal, add your favorite protein like grilled chicken, salmon, shrimp, sautéed tofu, or even crumbled turkey bacon.

For Salad

4 ounces baby spinach

4 ounces yellow grape tomatoes

20 pistachios, shelled and chopped

2 tablespoons crumbled goat cheese

For Dressing

1 teaspoon extra-virgin olive oil

1 medium scallion, thinly sliced

2 tablespoons orange juice

1 tablespoon white wine vinegar

1½ teaspoons golden monk fruit or brown sugar–style erythritol

1⁄16 teaspoon ground black pepper

1 Divide spinach between two medium serving bowls. Add rows of tomatoes, pistachios, and goat cheese evenly to bowls as well.

2 In a small saucepan over low to medium heat, heat oil. Add scallions and cook approximately 2 minutes until softened, swirling pan occasionally.

3 Add orange juice, vinegar, sweetener, and black pepper. Let simmer a few minutes until thoroughly heated. Pour dressing over salads and enjoy.

Creamy Feta Vinaigrette

Embracing the flavors of Greece, this dressing pairs well with hearty greens like spinach, field greens, or kale. Cover and refrigerate the leftovers up to 5 days. The stevia in this dressing is optional.

½ cup plain nonfat Greek yogurt

1 tablespoon lemon juice

1 tablespoon olive oil

1½ ounces crumbled feta cheese

2 teaspoons fresh mint

½ packet stevia

¼ teaspoon ground black pepper

Place all ingredients into a food processor or blender. Process until smooth. Chill before serving.

SERVES 11	
Per Serving (1 tablespoon):	
Calories	30
Fat	2g
Saturated Fat	1g
Cholesterol	5mg
Sodium	40mg
Carbohydrates	1g
Fiber	0g
Sugar	1g
Added Sugars	0g
Protein	2g

Fresh Peach-Mango Salsa

Fresh fruity salsas make wonderful toppings for grilled fish, meat, and poultry with the bonus of adding more plant foods to your meals.

1 cup peeled and diced mango

1 medium ripe peach, peeled, pitted, and diced

1 cup finely chopped red onion

1 cup peeled and diced cucumber

1 tablespoon balsamic vinegar

1 tablespoon lime juice

1 teaspoon chili powder

½ teaspoon ground cumin

1 tablespoon chopped fresh cilantro

1 tablespoon chopped fresh parsley

½ teaspoon kosher salt

In a medium bowl, mix all ingredients together. Chill at least 4 hours before serving.

SERVES 6	
Per Serving (½ cup):	
Calories	45
Fat	0g
Saturated Fat	0g
Cholesterol	0mg
Sodium	110mg
Carbohydrates	10g
Fiber	2g
Sugar	8g
Added Sugars	0g
Protein	1g

Peach, Corn, and Black Bean Salsa

SERVES 12

Per Serving (½ cup):

Calories	100
Fat	5g
Saturated Fat	1g
Cholesterol	0mg
Sodium	210mg
Carbohydrates	12g
Fiber	4g
Sugar	4g
Added Sugars	0g
Protein	3g

SERVING SUGGESTIONS

Serve this refreshing salsa to brighten your everyday meals. Use as a topping for chicken, fish, or burgers. Add to sandwiches or wraps with rotisserie chicken, pulled pork, canned tuna, plant-based burgers, or roasted vegetables.

Canned foods do most of the work in this delicious, gluten-free, vegan, and budget-friendly salsa. With a lovely mixture of sweet and mild spice, this will become a go-to for parties or any day.

3 medium tomatoes, seeded and diced

1 (15-ounce) can low-sodium black beans, drained and rinsed

1 (11-ounce) can corn kernels, drained and rinsed

1 cup canned peaches in juice, drained and diced (reserving 2 teaspoons liquid)

2 tablespoons chopped fresh cilantro

½ cup chopped scallions

¼ cup apple cider vinegar

¼ cup extra-virgin olive oil

2 teaspoons sriracha or hot sauce

⅛ teaspoon ground black pepper

⅛ teaspoon dried oregano

1 teaspoon kosher salt

1 In a large bowl, combine tomatoes, beans, corn, peaches, cilantro, and scallions. Set aside.

2 In a small bowl combine vinegar, oil, reserved peach juice, sriracha, black pepper, oregano, and salt, and whisk until emulsified.

3 Pour dressing over salsa and toss gently to combine. Serve.

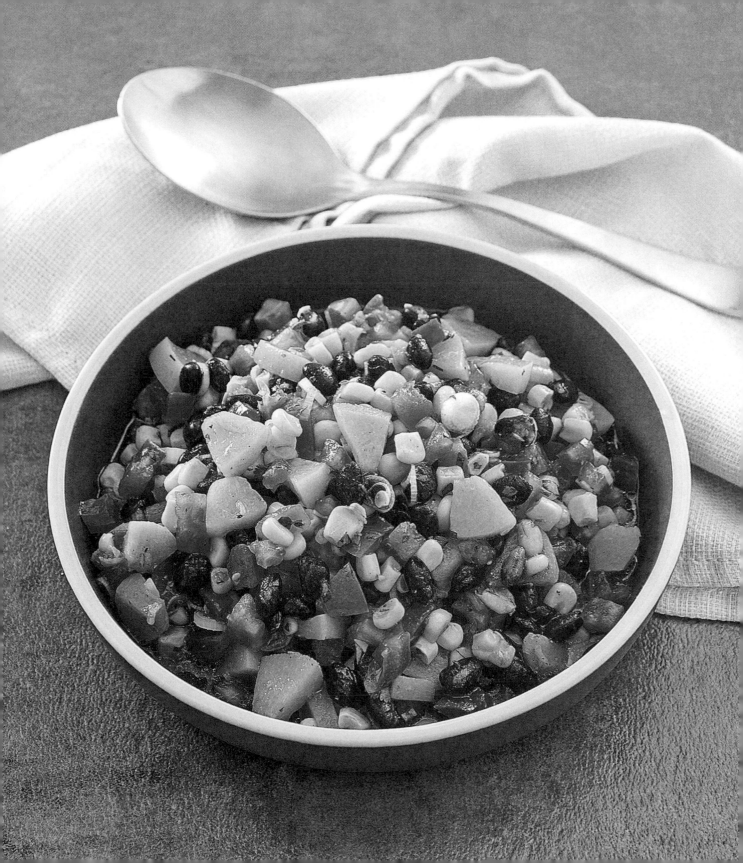

Greek Yogurt Balsamic Vinaigrette

Basic vinaigrettes can be high in fat and calories because the typical recipe uses a ratio of 2:1 oil to vinegar. This one reverses that ratio for a stronger flavor and adds Greek yogurt for creaminess and to help hold it together.

2 tablespoons extra-virgin olive oil

¼ cup balsamic vinegar

2 tablespoons nonfat plain Greek yogurt

1½ teaspoons honey

¹⁄₁₆ teaspoon kosher salt

¹⁄₁₆ teaspoon ground black pepper

In a small bowl, whisk together all ingredients. You could also shake well in a Mason jar. Serve. Cover and refrigerate any unused portion up to 5 days.

Power Salad

This salad is packed with nutritious superfoods like berries, kale, and nuts. The varied tastes and textures work well together for a hearty and filling plant-based meal. To effortlessly increase the protein, add canned salmon, tuna, or leftover rotisserie chicken.

1 (10-ounce) bag shaved Brussels sprouts

1 (5-ounce) package baby kale

6 cups chopped butter lettuce

1 cup fresh blueberries

1 cup chopped red apple

¼ cup dried cranberries

¼ cup chopped shelled pistachios

¼ cup Dijon Vinaigrette (see recipe in this chapter)

In a large bowl, combine Brussels sprouts, kale, lettuce, blueberries, apple, cranberries, and pistachios. Add dressing, toss, and serve.

Turkey-Avocado BLT Salad

Enjoy a healthier take on a classic flavor combo by turning your BLT into a salad. Subbing avocado in for the usual full-fat mayonnaise also gives a boost of heart-healthy monounsaturated fats.

2 slices uncured turkey bacon

3 ounces sliced reduced-sodium turkey breast

2 cups chopped salad greens (romaine or field greens)

½ cup halved grape tomatoes

¼ medium avocado, peeled, pitted, and diced

1 tablespoon Greek Yogurt Balsamic Vinaigrette (see recipe in this chapter)

1 Cook turkey bacon in microwave between paper towels according to package directions. Crumble and set aside.

2 Roll up turkey slices together into a tube shape and cut in even pieces so they look like spirals when turned on their sides.

3 Fill a medium bowl with salad greens. Add turkey, tomatoes, bacon, and diced avocado. Drizzle with dressing and serve.

SERVES 1	
Per Serving:	
Calories	280
Fat	13g
Saturated Fat	1.5g
Cholesterol	95mg
Sodium	770mg
Carbohydrates	14g
Fiber	6g
Sugar	7g
Added Sugars	1g
Protein	31g

Pumpkin Vinaigrette

Salad dressing is a little-known but terrific way to use the last bit of leftover pumpkin in the can. This flavor-packed dressing is low in sodium, vegan, and gluten-free too. Pumpkin has a unique ability to prevent your vinaigrette from "breaking," meaning it will allow the oil and vinegar to stay mixed. Plus, it adds a bit of sweetness so the dressing doesn't need sugar. It's a win-win.

1 tablespoon extra-virgin olive oil

2 tablespoons red wine vinegar

1½ teaspoons Dijon mustard

1½ teaspoons canned pumpkin purée

½ large clove garlic, peeled and finely chopped

⅛ teaspoon kosher salt

⅛ teaspoon ground black pepper

SERVES 2	
Per Serving (2 tablespoons):	
Calories	70
Fat	7g
Saturated Fat	1.5g
Cholesterol	0mg
Sodium	160mg
Carbohydrates	1g
Fiber	0g
Sugar	0g
Added Sugars	0g
Protein	0g

In a small bowl, whisk all ingredients together and then refrigerate to allow flavors to develop.

Israeli Salad

SERVES 4

Per Serving:

Calories	90
Fat	7g
Saturated Fat	1.5g
Cholesterol	0mg
Sodium	75mg
Carbohydrates	7g
Fiber	2g
Sugar	3g
Added Sugars	0g
Protein	2g

This traditional Middle Eastern dish is amazing alone, with added chickpeas and feta cheese for a plant-forward meal, or to bulk up the vegetable content of a wrap or pita. Add it to a burger, grilled fish, or poultry for a refreshing fiber boost.

1 large seedless English cucumber, diced with peel on

3 medium plum tomatoes, seeded and diced

3 medium scallions, diced

1 medium red or yellow bell pepper, seeded and diced

2 tablespoons extra-virgin olive oil

Juice of 1 medium lemon

¼ teaspoon kosher salt

⅛ teaspoon ground black pepper

¼ cup chopped fresh parsley

1 In a medium bowl, add cucumbers, tomatoes, scallions, and bell pepper.
2 In a small bowl, whisk oil, lemon juice, salt, and black pepper together. Pour over cucumber mixture and stir to combine.
3 Fold in parsley to gently combine and serve.

Sorghum Chicken and Vegetable Lettuce Wraps

Lettuce wraps are an easy way to pull together protein, grains, and vegetables in a light, quick meal. Swap out chicken for tuna, shrimp, or a vegetable burger so you will have a variety of fillings to choose from any day of the week.

½ cup cooked whole-grain sorghum

2 ounces grilled or rotisserie chicken, diced

⅓ cup grape or cherry tomatoes, halved

⅓ cup chopped red, orange, or yellow bell peppers

2 tablespoons Pumpkin Vinaigrette (see recipe in this chapter)

3 large romaine lettuce leaves

1 In a medium bowl, combine sorghum, chicken, tomatoes, and peppers.
2 Add dressing to sorghum mixture and gently combine.
3 Distribute sorghum mixture onto lettuce leaves and serve.

SERVES 1	
Per Serving:	
Calories	290
Fat	10g
Saturated Fat	2g
Cholesterol	50mg
Sodium	360mg
Carbohydrates	33g
Fiber	5g
Sugar	4g
Added Sugars	0g
Protein	21g

Cucumbers with Minted Yogurt

Light and refreshing, this yogurt-based dip is a lovely topping for beef, lamb, poultry, and fish as well as plant-based dishes like falafel.

1 cup plain nonfat Greek yogurt

1 medium clove garlic, peeled and finely chopped

¼ teaspoon ground cumin

1 teaspoon lemon zest

½ cup fresh mint, chopped

1 tablespoon lemon juice

¼ teaspoon salt

2 cups seeded and chopped cucumbers

1 In a blender or food processor, combine all ingredients except cucumbers and blend until smooth.
2 Add yogurt mixture to cucumbers and mix. Chill before serving.

SERVES 8	
Per Serving (¼ cup):	
Calories	25
Fat	0g
Saturated Fat	0g
Cholesterol	0mg
Sodium	85mg
Carbohydrates	2g
Fiber	0g
Sugar	1g
Added Sugars	0g
Protein	3g

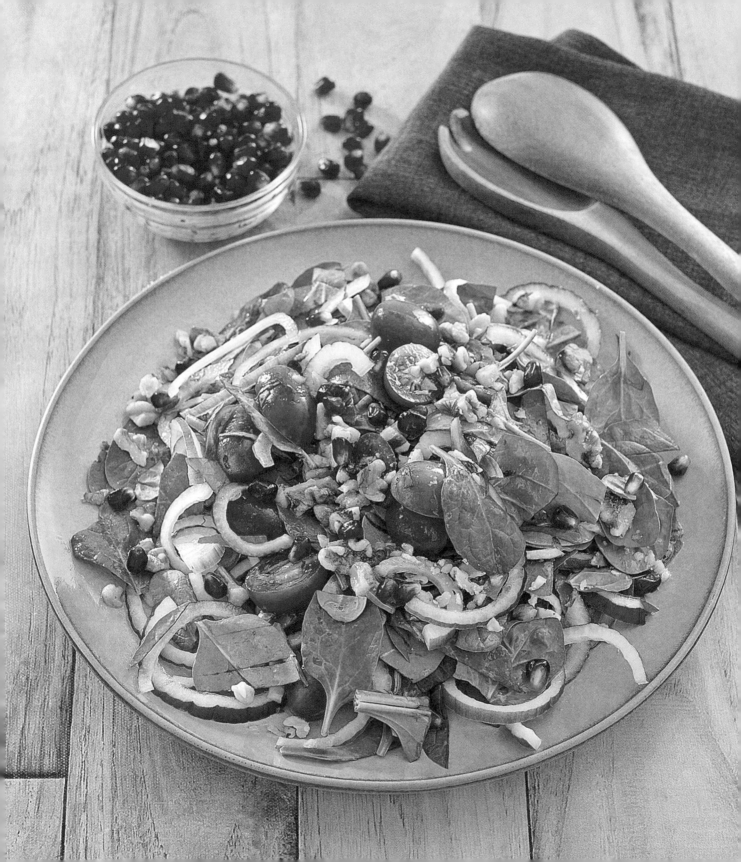

Spinach Salad with Pomegranate and Walnuts

Fruit and nuts are superb salad toppers, especially pomegranate seeds for their sweet and tangy crunch. Serve this as a starter or with grilled chicken, salmon, shrimp, steak, or tofu as an entrée salad.

1 pound fresh baby spinach, chopped

½ cup very thinly sliced red onion

8 ounces fresh grape tomatoes, halved

⅓ cup chopped walnuts, toasted

½ teaspoon kosher salt

¼ cup lemon juice

1½ tablespoons olive oil

¼ cup pomegranate seeds

1 Place spinach in a large bowl and add onion, tomatoes, and walnuts. Toss lightly to combine.

2 In a small bowl, whisk together salt, lemon juice, and oil. Drizzle dressing over salad and toss lightly.

3 Garnish salad with pomegranate seeds. Serve.

SERVES 6

Per Serving:

Calories	110
Fat	8g
Saturated Fat	1g
Cholesterol	0mg
Sodium	160mg
Carbohydrates	10g
Fiber	3g
Sugar	2g
Added Sugars	0g
Protein	4g

HOW TO PREPARE A POMEGRANATE

Rinse and score the pomegranate horizontally and vertically with a knife without cutting through to the seeds. Break it apart into quarters and submerge in a large bowl of water. With your hands under the water, separate the red seeds from the white pith that will float to the top. Scoop the floating pith out of the water and you should be left with the seeds. Drain in a strainer and keep in a covered container in the refrigerator for up to a week.

Dijon Vinaigrette

Once you make your own salad dressing, you'll never want to buy bottled dressing again! Use this recipe as a template and make it your own. Try different flavored vinegars, oils, and mustards or add herbs, minced scallions, crushed peppers, or citrus juice.

1 tablespoon Dijon mustard
¼ teaspoon kosher salt
¼ teaspoon ground black pepper
1½ tablespoons red wine vinegar
2 tablespoons extra-virgin olive oil
½ tablespoon water
½ packet stevia

In a small bowl, add all ingredients and use a wire whisk or fork to mix until emulsified. Store leftovers in an airtight container in the refrigerator up to 1 week.

SERVES 5	
Per Serving (1 tablespoon):	
Calories	50
Fat	6g
Saturated Fat	1g
Cholesterol	0mg
Sodium	180mg
Carbohydrates	0g
Fiber	0g
Sugar	0g
Added Sugars	0g
Protein	0g

Pomegranate Balsamic Vinaigrette

The deep flavors of pomegranate and balsamic vinegar are natural complements. Serve this dressing over simple greens with sliced fruit, grilled meat, and a little grated cheese.

3 tablespoons pomegranate juice
3 tablespoons balsamic vinegar
1 tablespoon olive oil
2 medium cloves garlic, peeled and minced
½ teaspoon dried Italian seasoning
⅛ teaspoon ground black pepper

1 In a small bowl, add all ingredients and whisk well to combine.
2 Use immediately or cover and refrigerate until ready to serve. If stored, whisk again before serving.

SERVES 4	
Per Serving (2 tablespoons):	
Calories	50
Fat	3.5g
Saturated Fat	0.5g
Cholesterol	0mg
Sodium	0mg
Carbohydrates	5g
Fiber	0g
Sugar	3g
Added Sugars	0g
Protein	0g

Vegan Caesar Salad Dressing

With undertones of garlic and lemon, this smooth and creamy dressing provides all of the flavor of the classic without the saturated fat. Toss with crisp romaine lettuce, your favorite chopped vegetables, and beans for extra protein.

¼ cup walnuts

¼ cup low-sodium vegetable broth

2 medium cloves garlic, peeled

1 tablespoon lemon juice

¾ teaspoon Dijon mustard

⅛ teaspoon kosher salt

⅛ teaspoon ground black pepper

1 Place all ingredients into a food processor. Pulse until smooth.
2 Serve. Store leftover dressing in refrigerator up to 5 days.

SERVES 4	
Per Serving (2 tablespoons):	
Calories	60
Fat	5g
Saturated Fat	0.5g
Cholesterol	0mg
Sodium	65mg
Carbohydrates	2g
Fiber	1g
Sugar	0g
Added Sugars	0g
Protein	1g

Spicy Lime, Cilantro, and Garlic Marinade

The most amazing citrusy, garlicky, spicy Southwestern taste imaginable. Spice up your meat, poultry, seafood, or tofu with this flavorful marinade.

2 teaspoons olive oil

½ cup finely chopped fresh cilantro

4 medium cloves garlic, peeled and minced

1 tablespoon red pepper flakes

¼ cup lime juice (from 2 medium limes)

1 In a medium mixing bowl, place oil. Add cilantro, garlic, and red pepper flakes and stir to combine.
2 Add lime juice and mix well.

MAKES 1 CUP	
Per Serving (¼ cup):	
Calories	35
Fat	2.5g
Saturated Fat	0g
Cholesterol	0mg
Sodium	0mg
Carbohydrates	3g
Fiber	1g
Sugar	0g
Added Sugars	0g
Protein	0g

Simple Autumn Salad

SERVES 4

Per Serving:

Calories	230
Fat	14g
Saturated Fat	2g
Cholesterol	0mg
Sodium	95mg
Carbohydrates	25g
Fiber	5g
Sugar	16g
Added Sugars	0g
Protein	4g

A tasty combination of red leaf lettuce, red onion, fruit, and walnuts in a light and tangy vinaigrette that you can enjoy any day of the week. If you are lucky enough to catch fresh figs during the short late summer or early fall, double the amount to 1 cup.

1 large head red leaf lettuce, torn into bite-sized pieces

1 medium pear, cored and thinly sliced

½ small red onion, peeled and thinly sliced

½ cup dried black Mission figs, chopped

⅓ cup chopped walnuts

2 tablespoons white balsamic vinegar

2 tablespoons olive oil

1 medium clove garlic, peeled and minced

¼ teaspoon ground black pepper

¼ teaspoon kosher salt

1 Place lettuce in a large bowl and add pear, onion, figs, and walnuts.
2 In a small bowl, add vinegar, oil, garlic, black pepper, and salt and whisk well to combine. Pour dressing over salad and toss to coat. Serve immediately.

Arugula with Pears and Red Wine Vinaigrette

The peppery taste of arugula is partnered with crisp, sweet pears and a tangy red wine vinaigrette. Add grilled chicken, chopped nuts, dried figs, and/or goat or feta cheese for a main-course salad.

8 cups baby arugula

2 medium pears, cored and thinly sliced

¼ cup red wine vinegar

2 tablespoons olive oil

1 medium clove garlic, peeled and minced

½ teaspoon dried oregano

¾ teaspoon Dijon mustard

¼ teaspoon ground black pepper

SERVES 4	
Per Serving:	
Calories	130
Fat	7g
Saturated Fat	1.5g
Cholesterol	0mg
Sodium	35mg
Carbohydrates	15g
Fiber	3g
Sugar	9g
Added Sugars	0g
Protein	1g

1 In a large bowl, place arugula and then add pears.
2 In a small bowl, add remaining ingredients and whisk well to combine. Pour over salad and toss to coat. Serve immediately.

Sesame Ginger Vinaigrette

Modeled after the dressings served at many Japanese restaurants, this low-sodium vinaigrette will have you craving salads like never before. A tiny bit of sugar will cut the acidity with only 1 gram of carbohydrate per serving.

¼ cup unflavored rice wine vinegar

1 tablespoon sesame oil

1 tablespoon minced fresh ginger

2 medium cloves garlic, peeled and minced

1 teaspoon sugar

¼ teaspoon ground black pepper

SERVES 3	
Per Serving (2 tablespoons):	
Calories	50
Fat	4.5g
Saturated Fat	0.5g
Cholesterol	0mg
Sodium	0mg
Carbohydrates	3g
Fiber	0g
Sugar	1g
Added Sugars	1g
Protein	0g

1 In a small microwave-safe bowl, add all ingredients and whisk well to combine. Microwave for 30 seconds, remove, and whisk well again.
2 Use immediately or refrigerate in a jar with a lid up to 5 days.

Deconstructed Spicy California Roll Salad

SERVES 2

Per Serving:

Calories	340
Fat	15g
Saturated Fat	2g
Cholesterol	15mg
Sodium	910mg
Carbohydrates	42g
Fiber	5g
Sugar	10g
Added Sugars	2g
Protein	10g

STICKY RICE

A standard California roll holds about 1 cup of rice, while this salad features ⅓ cup sticky rice. You can find sticky rice in a shelf-stable and microwave-safe container for great flavor while limiting the portion size to only one serving of carbohydrate per ⅓ cup.

This dish has all the authentic flavor of a spicy California roll from a sushi bar with way fewer carbs and fat. This huge salad is filling and delicious with no cooking necessary.

6 cups chopped romaine lettuce

⅓ large seedless English cucumber, peeled and sliced into matchsticks

4 imitation crab sticks, sliced into thin strips

½ medium ripe avocado, peeled, pitted, and sliced

⅔ cup cooked sticky rice

10 rectangular seaweed snack sheets, sliced into thin strips

¼ cup light mayonnaise

4 teaspoons sriracha

1 teaspoon lime juice

⅛ teaspoon sesame oil

1 Divide lettuce between two large serving bowls. Top each with half of cucumbers, crab, avocado, rice, and seaweed strips.

2 In a small bowl add mayonnaise, sriracha, lime juice, and oil and mix well to combine.

3 Transfer mayonnaise mixture into a sandwich-sized zip-top plastic bag and cut off one corner. Drizzle dressing onto both salads and serve.

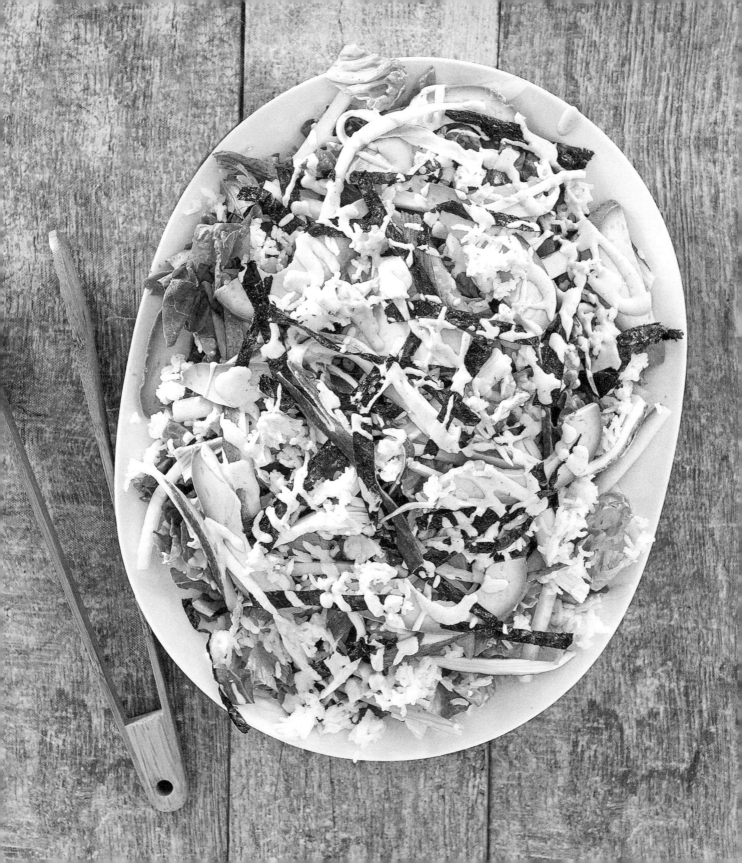

Strawberry Salsa

MAKES 2 CUPS

Per Serving (¼ cup):

Calories	25
Fat	0g
Saturated Fat	0g
Cholesterol	0mg
Sodium	0mg
Carbohydrates	6g
Fiber	1g
Sugar	4g
Added Sugars	1g
Protein	1g

A truly stellar salsa made from fresh strawberries. The cinnamon adds depth to the triumvirate of spicy, sweet, and savory flavors.

2 cups chopped fresh strawberries

1 small yellow or orange bell pepper, seeded and chopped

1 medium jalapeño pepper, seeded and minced

2 medium cloves garlic, peeled and minced

2 tablespoons chopped fresh cilantro

Juice of 1 medium lemon

2 teaspoons honey

1 teaspoon minced fresh ginger

½ teaspoon ground cinnamon

½ teaspoon ground cumin

1 In a medium bowl, add all ingredients and stir well to combine.
2 Serve immediately or cover and refrigerate until ready to serve.

Homemade High-Fiber Bread Crumbs

SERVES 12

Per Serving (¼ cup):

Calories	25
Fat	0g
Saturated Fat	0g
Cholesterol	0mg
Sodium	85mg
Carbohydrates	9g
Fiber	5g
Sugar	1g
Added Sugars	0g
Protein	1g

Homemade bread crumbs are so simple to make. They're lower in sodium, carbs, and calories, and much higher in fiber when starting with high-fiber bread.

8 slices light, high-fiber bread (40–50 calories per slice)

1 Preheat oven to 300°F.
2 Place bread slices on a large baking sheet and bake 10 minutes, flip over, and bake an additional 5–10 minutes until crisp but not browned.
3 Let cool for several minutes and place in a food processor, blending until you have the consistency of panko-style bread crumbs.
4 Store in an airtight container.

CHAPTER 10
Snacks and Desserts

Pumpkin Chip Energy Bites

These bite-sized snacks are packed with fiber, whole grains, and omega-3 fatty acids thanks to fiber cereal, oats, and flax seeds. Pop a bite to get your fiber on the go.

⅔ cup high-fiber cereal, such as Fiber One

¼ cup old-fashioned oats

¼ cup ground flaxseed meal

¼ cup natural peanut butter, no added sugar

¼ cup canned pure pumpkin

2½ tablespoons sugar-free maple syrup

½ teaspoon vanilla extract

1½ teaspoons pumpkin pie spice

¼ cup sugar-free chocolate chips

1 Place all ingredients except chocolate chips into a food processor. Blend until a ball of dough forms. If the dough is dry, add a little water, 1 teaspoon at a time.

2 Transfer dough to a medium bowl and fold in chocolate chips.

3 Cover and refrigerate 20 minutes. Remove from refrigerator and use a small scoop (about 1 rounded tablespoon) of dough and roll in your hands to form a ball.

4 Enjoy immediately or refrigerate the extras in a container with a lid for several days.

Cranberry Banana Whole-Grain Muffins

These Cranberry Banana Whole-Grain Muffins are bursting with fresh cranberries and rich in whole-grain goodness, making them a yummy snack for the whole family.

1 large egg

1 teaspoon vanilla extract

3 tablespoons extra-light olive oil or canola oil

2 tablespoons plain nonfat Greek yogurt

½ cup granular monk fruit, erythritol, or stevia

½ teaspoon salt

3 medium ripe bananas, mashed

1½ cups white whole-wheat flour

1 teaspoon baking soda

1 teaspoon baking powder

¾ cup fresh or frozen whole cranberries

1 Preheat oven to 350°F. Line a twelve-cup muffin tin with liners or spray with nonstick cooking spray.

2 In a large mixing bowl, beat egg with a fork. Add vanilla, oil, yogurt, monk fruit, and salt and mix well. Stir in bananas.

3 In a medium bowl, combine flour, baking soda, and baking powder.

4 Slowly add dry ingredients to wet, stirring to combine, avoiding overmixing. Fold in cranberries.

5 Fill muffin cups about three-quarters full with batter. Bake approximately 20 minutes until toothpick comes out clean. Cool for a few minutes before removing from pan.

SERVES 12

Per Serving (1 muffin):

Calories	120
Fat	4g
Saturated Fat	0.5g
Cholesterol	15mg
Sodium	240mg
Carbohydrates	27g
Fiber	5g
Sugar	4g
Added Sugars	0g
Protein	3g

SUBSTITUTE WHITE WHOLE-WHEAT FLOUR IN BAKED GOODS

White whole-wheat flour is fabulous for baking because it has whole-grain nutrition without the tannins that can make regular whole-wheat flour bitter. It comes from a different species of wheat and though white is in the name, it refers to the color, not the nutritional value.

Sugar-Free Chocolate Chip Zucchini Bread Squares

SERVES 16

Per Serving:

Calories	60
Fat	1.5g
Saturated Fat	0.5g
Cholesterol	0mg
Sodium	150mg
Carbohydrates	16g
Fiber	3g
Sugar	1g
Added Sugars	0g
Protein	3g

SQUARES VERSUS SLICES

Baking in a brownie pan versus a loaf pan cuts cooking time in half and allows for easier slicing into smaller servings. Enjoy one for a snack or on top of cottage cheese or Greek yogurt for breakfast.

Quick breads are usually loaded with oil and sugar, but not these zucchini bread squares. Using oats as flour ups the blood sugar–stabilizing soluble fiber, and Greek yogurt and zucchini add lots of moisture without extra fat.

2 cups old-fashioned oats

½ cup granular erythritol or monk fruit

2 tablespoons golden monk fruit or brown sugar–style erythritol

1 tablespoon ground cinnamon

⅛ teaspoon ground nutmeg

2 teaspoons baking powder

½ teaspoon baking soda

⅛ teaspoon salt

1 teaspoon vanilla extract

½ cup liquid egg whites

⅓ cup plain nonfat Greek yogurt

1 medium (about 10 ounces) zucchini, stemmed and grated

3 tablespoons sugar-free chocolate chips, divided

1 Preheat oven to 350°F. Line a 9" × 9" brownie pan with parchment paper. Spray with nonstick cooking spray and set aside.

2 In a food processor, blend oats until you have a coarse flour. Add remaining ingredients except zucchini and chocolate chips and process until smooth. Stir in zucchini and 1 tablespoon chocolate chips.

3 Pour batter into pan and top with remaining 2 tablespoons chocolate chips. Bake about 30 minutes. (This recipe works better when just underdone.)

4 Let cool at least 10 minutes before slicing. Cut into sixteen squares and serve. Store any uneaten squares in the refrigerator.

Skinny Banana Bread Squares

Savor the flavors of banana and chocolate in these snack-sized squares that are perfectly portioned for breakfast, snacks, or dessert.

2 cups old-fashioned oats

3 tablespoons golden monk fruit or brown sugar–style erythritol

2 tablespoons granular monk fruit or erythritol

1 teaspoon ground cinnamon

1 teaspoon baking powder

1 teaspoon baking soda

½ teaspoon salt

4 medium ripe bananas

1 large egg

1 tablespoon vanilla extract

¼ cup plain nonfat Greek yogurt

1½ tablespoons mini chocolate chips

SERVES 16

Per Serving:

Calories	80
Fat	1.5g
Saturated Fat	0.5g
Cholesterol	10mg
Sodium	190mg
Carbohydrates	18g
Fiber	2g
Sugar	4g
Added Sugars	0g
Protein	2g

1 Preheat oven to 350°F. Line a 9" × 9" brownie pan with parchment paper and spray with nonstick cooking spray.

2 Pulse oats in a food processor to consistency of a coarse flour. Add remaining ingredients except chocolate chips and blend until smooth.

3 Pour batter into pan, smooth out, and top with chocolate chips.

4 Bake 30 minutes or until toothpick inserted in center comes out clean. (This recipe works better when just underdone.)

5 Let squares cool, then cut into sixteen pieces and serve. Store any uneaten squares in refrigerator.

Sugar-Free Black Bean Avocado Brownie Bites

TIPS

While many recipes can use sweeteners interchangeably, this one works best with monk fruit or erythritol, not stevia, for the best flavor and texture. If you don't have a silicone mini muffin tray, bake regular brownies by lining a 9" × 9" brownie pan with parchment paper. Pour in batter and bake at 350°F for 35–40 minutes.

No one will ever guess these decadent brownie bites are loaded with nutrient-rich ingredients without any grains, gluten, or added sugars.

1 (15-ounce) can low-sodium black beans, drained and rinsed

3 large eggs

¼ cup plain nonfat Greek yogurt

½ cup unsweetened cocoa powder

¾ cup granular monk fruit or erythritol

¼ teaspoon salt

1 teaspoon baking powder

1 teaspoon vanilla extract

1 medium avocado, peeled, pitted, and sliced

½ cup sugar-free chocolate chips

1 Preheat oven to 350°F.
2 Place all ingredients except chocolate chips into a food processor and blend until smooth. Stir in chocolate chips.
3 Spray twenty-four silicone mini muffin cups with nonstick cooking spray and fill cups about three-quarters full with batter. Bake 19 minutes or until toothpick inserted in comes out clean. (This recipe works better when just underdone.)
4 Let bites cool before removing from silicone and serving.

Roasted Pears with Dried Plums and Pistachios

These Roasted Pears with Dried Plums and Pistachios are super versatile with a great mix of textures you can enjoy for breakfast, snacks, or dessert. Top one with cottage cheese or Greek yogurt to pack your breakfast with protein and fiber.

2 medium ripe pears

4 medium dried plums, diced

30 pistachios, shelled and crushed

1 teaspoon ground cinnamon

2 teaspoons pure maple syrup

1 Preheat oven or toaster oven to 350°F. Line a small baking tray with foil.

2 Slice pears in half from stem down, then take a thin slice off the bottom edge of halves so pears lie flat and don't wobble on tray. Gently scoop core and seeds out of pear center leaving room for the filling.

3 Fill pears evenly with dried plums and pistachios. Sprinkle on cinnamon.

4 Drizzle each pear half with ½ teaspoon syrup. Bake 25 minutes or until pear is soft but not mushy. Serve.

SERVES 4

Per Serving (½ pear):

Calories	110
Fat	2g
Saturated Fat	0g
Cholesterol	0mg
Sodium	25mg
Carbohydrates	22g
Fiber	4g
Sugar	13g
Added Sugars	2g
Protein	1g

PURE MAPLE SYRUP

The tiny bit of pure maple syrup in this recipe only adds 2 grams of carbohydrates and brings a lot of flavor. You can also substitute honey or sorghum syrup, which resembles molasses. Top the extras with cottage cheese or plain Greek yogurt for breakfast.

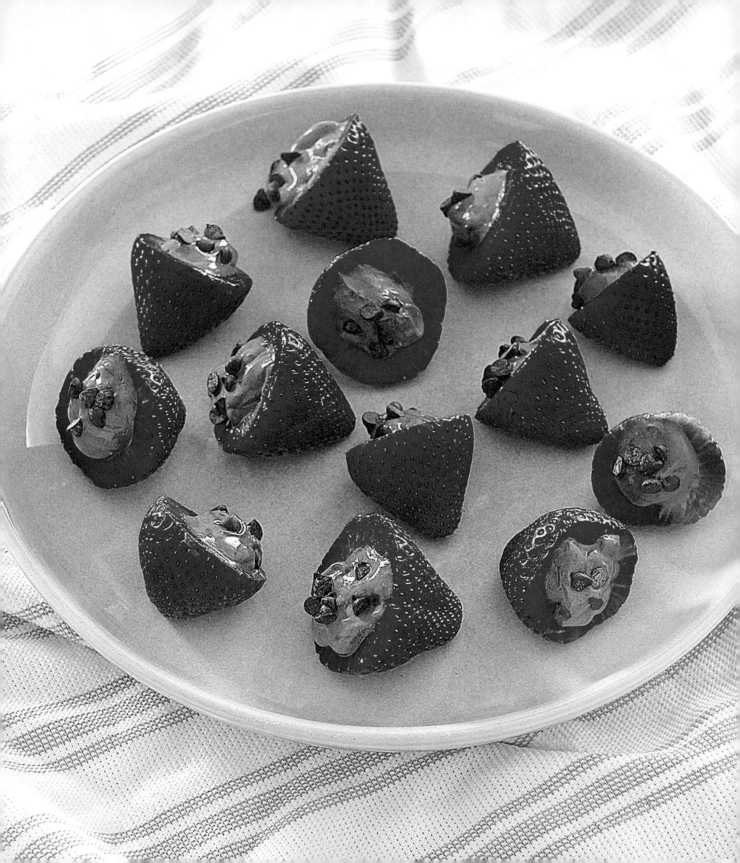

Chocolate Mousse–Stuffed Strawberries

These decadent Chocolate Mousse–Stuffed Strawberries are low in sugar, gluten-free, vegan, and have only 70 calories per serving! A perfect dessert for any occasion.

3 ounces soft/silken tofu, patted dry

2 tablespoons unsweetened cocoa powder

2 packets stevia

16 medium strawberries, stemmed and hulled

1 tablespoon mini vegan chocolate chips

1 In a blender or small food processor, add tofu, cocoa powder, and stevia. Blend until smooth (will make about ¼ cup plus 2 tablespoons).

2 Transfer mixture into a zip-top plastic bag or pastry bag. Cut off corner of zip-top bag and pipe cocoa mixture into each strawberry.

3 Top each with a few mini chocolate chips. Serve.

SERVES 4

Per Serving (4 strawberries):

Calories	70
Fat	2g
Saturated Fat	0.5g
Cholesterol	0mg
Sodium	10mg
Carbohydrates	12g
Fiber	3g
Sugar	7g
Added Sugars	2g
Protein	3g

TIPS

Some may prefer the mousse a bit sweeter, so taste it first and add extra stevia if necessary. Remember that it will pick up sweetness from the berries and chocolate chips. To make the filling and serving process easier, cut off the very bottom tip of the strawberry to create a flat surface and allow it to stand up.

Chocolate-Dipped Fruit

SERVES 3	
Per Serving:	
Calories	210
Fat	9g
Saturated Fat	6g
Cholesterol	0mg
Sodium	0mg
Carbohydrates	36g
Fiber	6g
Sugar	22g
Added Sugars	9g
Protein	3g

Chocolate-covered fruit should be much more than a once-a-year Valentine's Day treat. Making your own at home is so simple, yet it feels so fancy. If you wish to lower the sugar content further, choose a sugar-free variety of chocolate chips.

⅓ cup dark chocolate chips

6 large strawberries

1 medium pear, cored and sliced into 6 pieces

1 medium under-ripe banana, peeled and sliced into 1"-thick pieces

1 Fill a tall, narrow pot with about 2" water and heat to a simmer (not boiling).

2 Place a medium heatproof glass or metal bowl on top of pot to make a double boiler. Holding bowl with a potholder or oven mitt, add chocolate and stir with a wooden or silicone spoon until melted and smooth.

3 Line a medium baking pan with parchment paper. Using fingers or a skewer, dip fruit pieces halfway into chocolate to coat and place on pan.

4 Place pan in refrigerator to allow chocolate to harden. Results are best if served the same day.

Chocolate Haystacks

Dessert with benefits? Typically made with fried Chinese-style noodles, the whole family will go crazy for these no-bake haystacks made better for you with high-fiber cereal.

12 ounces (approximately 2 cups) chocolate chips, any flavor

4 cups high-fiber cereal, such as Fiber One

1 Fill a tall, narrow pot with about 2" water and heat to a simmer (not boiling).

2 Place a medium heatproof glass or metal bowl on top of pot to make a double boiler. Holding bowl with a potholder or oven mitt, add chocolate and stir with a wooden or silicone spoon until melted and smooth.

3 Gently fold cereal into chocolate until thoroughly coated. Remove bowl from heat.

4 Line a medium baking sheet with parchment paper or a silicone liner. Using a disposable glove or two spoons, drop haystacks (about 1 rounded tablespoon each) onto baking sheet.

5 Let cool at least 10 minutes or put in refrigerator or freezer to cool faster before serving. Store uneaten portions in an airtight container.

MAKES 48 HAYSTACKS

Per Serving:

Calories	45
Fat	2g
Saturated Fat	1.5g
Cholesterol	0mg
Sodium	15mg
Carbohydrates	9g
Fiber	3g
Sugar	4g
Added Sugars	4g
Protein	1g

CUSTOMIZE YOUR HAYSTACKS

These are so much fun to customize for any occasion. Simply add toppings to haystacks before they cool. Think of dried or freeze-dried fruit pieces or sprinkles of all different colors to serve for various holidays. You can reduce the sugar by using sugar-free chocolate chips, though they don't melt as well and you may need to add a little bit of oil during the melting process for a smoother texture.

Cranberry Pistachio Granola Bar Squares

SERVES 16

Per Serving:

Calories	100
Fat	4.5g
Saturated Fat	0.5g
Cholesterol	0mg
Sodium	70mg
Carbohydrates	12g
Fiber	1g
Sugar	6g
Added Sugars	6g
Protein	3g

VARIATIONS

Once you have the base recipe, you can easily play around with it. One of the best things about these bars is their versatility. You can use any type of nuts; think almonds, walnuts, cashews, or pecans. Almost any dried fruit works well, too, like cherries, dates, raisins, or apricots. Use your imagination!

Snack smart with these tasty, chewy, crunchy squares that are a satisfying treat containing heart-healthy fats and fiber from nutrient-dense whole foods. Plus, they are missing the unwanted ingredients you will find in most commercial granola bars.

1 cup old-fashioned oats

¼ cup shelled pumpkin seeds

2 tablespoons ground flaxseed meal

¼ cup roughly chopped shelled pistachios

¼ cup chopped dried cranberries

¾ cup unsweetened whole-grain puffed rice cereal

¼ cup creamy natural peanut butter, no added sugar

¼ cup raw honey

½ teaspoon vanilla extract

¼ teaspoon salt

1. Preheat oven to 350°F. Spray a 9" × 9" square brownie pan with nonstick cooking spray and set aside.
2. On a medium rimmed baking sheet, combine oats, pumpkin seeds, and flaxseed. Bake 3 minutes.
3. Add pistachios and continue baking an additional 2–3 minutes, taking care not to burn them.
4. Remove oat mixture from oven and place in a large bowl. Add cranberries and puffed rice cereal, toss, and set aside.
5. In a small saucepan over medium-low heat, combine peanut butter, honey, vanilla, and salt. Cook while stirring gently until bubbly, about 3 minutes.
6. Remove from heat and pour peanut butter mixture over oat mixture, stirring well with a large spoon or spatula until thoroughly combined.
7. Transfer to prepared pan and press with a spatula until mixture is flat and even. Place in freezer 10–15 minutes to firm up.
8. Cut into sixteen squares and enjoy. Refrigerate leftovers in a tightly sealed container up to 5 days.

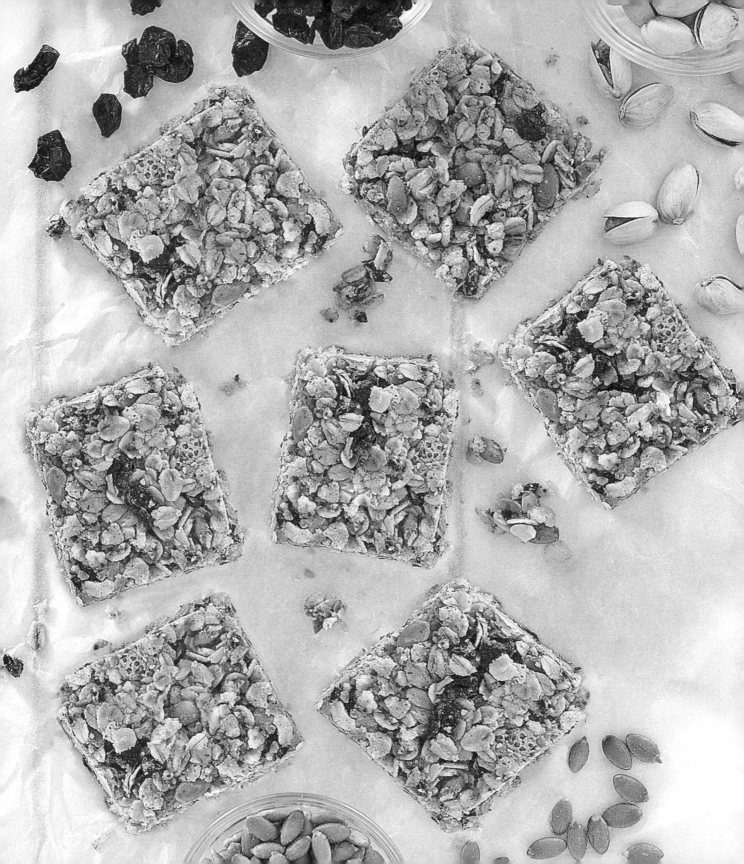

Chocolate Chip Cookie Dough Dip

SERVES 8

Per Serving (¼ cup):

Calories	160
Fat	7g
Saturated Fat	2.5g
Cholesterol	0mg
Sodium	150mg
Carbohydrates	20g
Fiber	5g
Sugar	1g
Added Sugars	0g
Protein	5g

ADJUSTMENTS

Feel free to substitute chickpeas for the white beans if you have them on hand. If you prefer a thinner dip, add unsweetened nut milk 1 teaspoon at a time and blend until the desired consistency is achieved.

No one will believe that this delicious dip is made from white beans! Enjoy by itself with a spoon or as a dip for apple slices, strawberries, or graham crackers.

1 (15-ounce) can cannellini beans, drained and rinsed

¼ cup natural creamy peanut butter

¼ cup old-fashioned oats

¼ teaspoon baking powder

¼ teaspoon ground cinnamon

¼ teaspoon kosher salt

¼ cup sugar-free maple syrup

2 tablespoons brown sugar–style erythritol or golden monk fruit

1 tablespoon vanilla extract

⅓ cup sugar-free chocolate chips

1 Place all ingredients except chocolate chips into a food processor. Blend until smooth, scraping down the sides as needed.

2 Stir in chocolate chips and serve. Refrigerate leftovers in a tightly sealed container for a few days.

Chocolate Doughnuts with Vanilla Glaze

No one will guess these indulgent treats are low in sugar! Double the recipe for a crowd or if you want to freeze extras without the glaze.

½ cup white whole-wheat flour

2 tablespoons unsweetened cocoa powder

½ plus ⅛ teaspoon baking powder

⅛ teaspoon salt

¼ cup granular monk fruit or erythritol

2 tablespoons liquid egg whites

¾ teaspoon vanilla extract, divided

½ cup 1% milk, divided

2 tablespoons mini chocolate chips

⅓ cup confectioners' sugar alternative (made with erythritol or stevia)

SERVES 6	
Per Serving:	
Calories	80
Fat	2g
Saturated Fat	1g
Cholesterol	0mg
Sodium	135mg
Carbohydrates	29g
Fiber	4g
Sugar	4g
Added Sugars	3g
Protein	3g

1 Preheat oven to 350°F. Spray a six-hole doughnut pan with non-stick cooking spray.

2 In a medium bowl, add flour, cocoa powder, baking powder, and salt and stir.

3 In a small bowl, whisk monk fruit and egg whites, then add ½ teaspoon vanilla and all but 2 teaspoons milk. Whisk until smooth.

4 Combine wet ingredients with dry ingredients and stir to combine; do not overmix. Gently fold in chocolate chips.

5 Spoon mixture evenly into doughnut pan and bake 10–15 minutes until done.

6 While doughnuts are cooking, prepare glaze. In a small bowl, mix confectioners' sugar alternative, remaining 2 teaspoons milk, and remaining ¼ teaspoon vanilla.

7 When doughnuts are done, transfer to a medium plate. Cool for a few minutes and then dip into glaze. Serve.

Roasted Everything Chickpeas

This protein- and fiber-rich crunchy snack is available in many different flavors in the supermarket, but why not make your own for a fraction of the cost? Use any seasoning you want, savory or sweet. Everything bagel seasoning is so flavorful you'll make these again and again.

1 (15-ounce) can low-sodium chickpeas, drained and rinsed

1 tablespoon olive oil

1 teaspoon everything bagel seasoning

1 Preheat oven to 425°F. Line a medium baking sheet with parchment paper.

2 Dry chickpeas well with a clean dish towel and discard any loose skins that separate. Place chickpeas in a medium bowl, coat with oil, and toss. Transfer to prepared baking sheet and bake 20–22 minutes, stirring after 10 minutes.

3 Remove from oven and sprinkle with bagel seasoning. Once cool, store leftovers in an airtight container.

Apple Raisin Matzo Kugel

A healthy dessert that also makes a great side dish or breakfast. Top with cottage cheese or Greek yogurt to up the protein for a balanced breakfast or with a dollop of light vanilla ice cream for a delicious snack or after-dinner treat.

3 sheets whole-wheat matzo

2 cups water

3 medium apples such as Honeycrisp or Gala, cored and thinly sliced

1 tablespoon lemon juice

3 tablespoons unsalted butter, melted

¼ cup golden monk fruit or brown sugar–style erythritol

½ cup raisins

3 large egg whites

⅛ teaspoon kosher salt

1½ teaspoons ground cinnamon, plus more to sprinkle on top

1 Preheat oven to 375°F. Spray a 9" × 13" metal baking dish with nonstick cooking spray and set aside.

2 Place matzo in an 8" square baking pan. Pour water into pan and set aside to rehydrate.

3 When soft, drain matzo and squeeze out excess water.

4 Place matzo into a medium bowl and add remaining ingredients. Stir well to combine.

5 Pour mixture into baking dish and sprinkle with additional cinnamon. Place on middle rack in oven and bake 15–20 minutes until apples are soft.

6 Remove from oven and place on a wire rack to cool. Cut into portions and serve warm or cool.

SERVES 8	
Per Serving:	
Calories	160
Fat	4.5g
Saturated Fat	2.5g
Cholesterol	10mg
Sodium	40mg
Carbohydrates	30g
Fiber	4g
Sugar	14g
Added Sugars	0g
Protein	3g

Whole-Wheat Strawberry Corn Muffins

Fabulous vegan muffins with the taste and texture of traditional muffins. The combination of plump moist berries and subtle crunch of cornmeal is irresistible.

1 cup white whole-wheat flour

½ cup cornmeal

½ cup granular monk fruit, erythritol, or stevia

2 teaspoons baking powder

⅛ teaspoon salt

1 cup chopped fresh strawberries

1 cup unsweetened nondairy milk, such as almond, cashew, or oat

3 tablespoons canola oil

2 teaspoons vanilla extract

1 Preheat oven to 375°F. Line a twelve-cup muffin tin with liners or spray with nonstick cooking spray and set aside.
2 In a large bowl, add flour, cornmeal, monk fruit, baking powder, and salt and whisk well to combine.
3 Add strawberries, nondairy milk, oil, and vanilla and stir until incorporated.
4 Fill muffin cups roughly two-thirds full. Place muffin tin on middle rack in oven and bake 18–20 minutes.
5 Remove from oven and place on a wire rack to cool. Serve.

Perfect Corn Bread

This foolproof corn bread strikes the ideal balance between sweet and savory.

1 cup cornmeal

¾ cup white whole-wheat flour

2 teaspoons baking powder

⅓ cup granular stevia, erythritol, or monk fruit

¼ teaspoon salt

1 cup 1% milk

1 large egg white

¼ cup olive oil

1 teaspoon vanilla extract

1 Preheat oven to 425°F. Spray an 8" baking pan with nonstick cooking spray and set aside.

2 In a medium bowl, add all ingredients and stir well to combine. Pour batter into prepared pan.

3 Place pan on middle rack in oven and bake 17–20 minutes. Take care not to overbake.

4 Remove from oven and place on a wire rack to cool. Cut into squares and serve.

SERVES 16

Per Serving:

Calories	100
Fat	4g
Saturated Fat	0.5g
Cholesterol	0mg
Sodium	125mg
Carbohydrates	17g
Fiber	3g
Sugar	1g
Added Sugars	0g
Protein	2g

FABULOUS FAT-FREE CORN BREAD!

Make an equally delicious fat-free version of this corn bread by substituting ¼ cup unsweetened applesauce for the oil and skim milk for the low-fat milk. Add ½ cup frozen corn to the batter for an added treat.

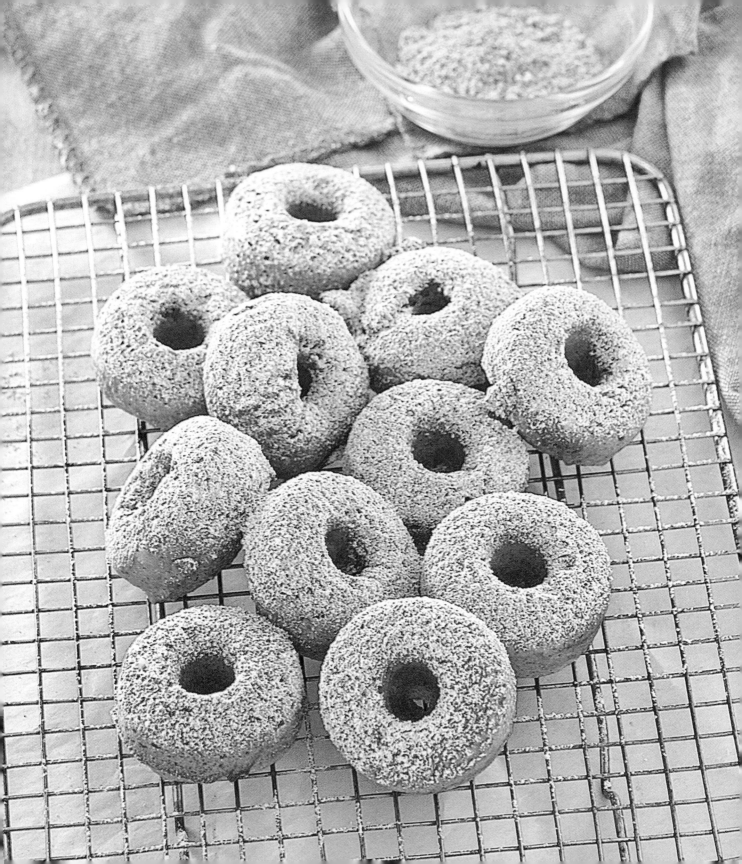

Baked Cinnamon Doughnuts

The essence of cinnamon and sugar is so comforting. These low-fat, whole-grain doughnuts are so easy to make and enjoy whenever the craving hits.

1 cup white whole-wheat flour

⅓ cup granular erythritol

1 teaspoon baking powder

1 teaspoon ground cinnamon, divided

½ cup 1% milk

½ teaspoon vanilla extract

1 large egg white

1 tablespoon confectioners' sugar alternative (made with erythritol)

1 Preheat oven to 425°F. Spray a six-hole doughnut pan with non-stick cooking spray and set aside.

2 In a medium bowl, add flour, granular erythritol, baking powder, and ½ teaspoon cinnamon and whisk to combine.

3 Add milk, vanilla, and egg white and beat well.

4 Spoon batter into prepared doughnut pan, filling about two-thirds full. Place pan on middle rack in oven. Bake 10–13 minutes until tops are no longer moist.

5 Remove pan from oven and let rest a few minutes before gently removing doughnuts from pan.

6 In a small bowl, combine erythritol confectioners' sugar alternative and remaining ½ teaspoon cinnamon and mix. Dip doughnuts into mixture and serve immediately or place on a wire rack to cool.

SERVES 6	
Per Serving:	
Calories	90
Fat	0.5g
Saturated Fat	0g
Cholesterol	0mg
Sodium	125mg
Carbohydrates	29g
Fiber	6g
Sugar	1g
Added Sugars	0g
Protein	4g

DOUGHNUT PANS

Doughnuts pans, like muffins tins, are trays with special circular cutouts for batter. In the case of a doughnut pan, however, the rounds are wide and shallow, with a small tubular protrusion in the center for the doughnut hole. Doughnut pans are inexpensive and will last for years if gently hand washed. Select a pan with a non-stick coating to minimize the need for added oil. Doughnut pans are available in metal and silicone. The cooking time may vary by type of pan used.

Sweet and Spicy Roasted Almonds

Roasted nuts are a delicious, nutritious snack or crunchy addition to salads, cereal, yogurt, trail mix, and much more. Store leftovers in a sealed container for up to 2 weeks.

SERVES 8	
Per Serving:	
Calories	180
Fat	15g
Saturated Fat	1g
Cholesterol	0mg
Sodium	40mg
Carbohydrates	7g
Fiber	4g
Sugar	1g
Added Sugars	0g
Protein	6g

1 large egg white

⅛ teaspoon ground cayenne pepper

1 teaspoon ground cinnamon

1½ tablespoons brown sugar–style erythritol

¼ teaspoon kosher salt

2 cups whole unsalted almonds

1 Preheat oven to 350°F.
2 In a medium bowl, whisk egg white until frothy. Stir in cayenne, cinnamon, erythritol, and salt.
3 Add almonds and toss to coat with egg white mixture.
4 Pour almonds onto a medium baking sheet and bake 10 minutes, stir, and bake an additional 8–10 minutes, taking care not to burn almonds in the last few minutes.
5 Remove from oven and let cool. Serve.

Frozen Yogurt Bark

When the temperature goes up, we all crave cool, refreshing snacks. Frozen yogurt bark is a super easy way to enjoy a high-protein, low-sugar frozen snack. Swap in any nut or dried fruit for endless flavor combinations.

1 (5.3-ounce) container low-sugar vanilla nonfat Greek yogurt

2 tablespoons dried cranberries

30 pistachios, shelled and chopped

1 Line a medium baking sheet with parchment paper and spread yogurt out in a thin layer.
2 Top with cranberries and pistachios. Place in the freezer 20 minutes.
3 Break into pieces and serve. Store leftovers in freezer in a zip-top plastic bag or a container with lid. Defrost a few minutes before eating for the best texture.

SERVES 2	
Per Serving:	
Calories	110
Fat	4g
Saturated Fat	0g
Cholesterol	5mg
Sodium	110mg
Carbohydrates	13g
Fiber	1g
Sugar	10g
Added Sugars	5g
Protein	8g

Homemade Banana "Nice" Cream

This dessert contains only one ingredient: bananas. Yet when frozen and puréed, the crystallized fruit mimics the look, taste, and texture of ice cream so perfectly, it's almost magic. For ease of preparation, peel and slice the bananas prior to freezing them. Switch up the flavor by adding cocoa powder, vanilla extract, or powdered peanut butter. Create a sundae by topping with a few chocolate chips, chopped nuts, and a small amount of whipped cream for a special treat.

4 medium ripe bananas, sliced and frozen

1 Remove bananas from freezer. Place slices into a blender or food processor and pulse until smooth.
2 Scoop mixture out and serve immediately.

SERVES 4	
Per Serving:	
Calories	110
Fat	0g
Saturated Fat	0g
Cholesterol	0mg
Sodium	0mg
Carbohydrates	27g
Fiber	3g
Sugar	14g
Added Sugars	0g
Protein	1g

Pumpkin Chocolate Chip Muffins

SERVES 10

Per Serving:

Calories	120
Fat	6g
Saturated Fat	2g
Cholesterol	0mg
Sodium	135mg
Carbohydrates	21g
Fiber	3g
Sugar	1g
Added Sugars	0g
Protein	3g

Moist, dense, and pumpkin rich, these muffins make for a yummy breakfast, snack, or dessert. Substitute chopped nuts or dried fruit for the chocolate chips if desired.

1 cup pumpkin purée

½ cup brown sugar–style erythritol

1 large egg white

2 tablespoons canola oil

2 tablespoons plain nonfat Greek yogurt

1 teaspoon vanilla extract

2 teaspoons baking powder

½ teaspoon ground cinnamon

½ teaspoon pumpkin pie spice

1 cup white whole-wheat flour

⅓ cup sugar-free semisweet chocolate chips

1 Preheat oven to 400°F. Spray ten muffin tin cups with nonstick cooking spray and set aside.

2 In a large bowl, place pumpkin, erythritol, egg white, oil, yogurt, and vanilla and stir well to combine. Add remaining ingredients and mix until incorporated.

3 Spoon batter into muffin cups, filling each cup about two-thirds full. Place pan on middle rack in oven and bake 17–20 minutes.

4 Remove from oven and place muffins on a wire rack to cool. Serve.

Amaretto Roasted Peaches

These sweet summer peaches are a heavenly treat. For an extra rich dessert, top your peach with fresh whipped cream or a dollop of vanilla frozen yogurt. Enjoy any leftovers for breakfast with Greek yogurt, cottage cheese, or ricotta.

3 large ripe to very ripe peaches, halved and pitted

2 tablespoons amaretto liquor

2 tablespoons rum

⅛ teaspoon vanilla extract

¼ cup old-fashioned oats, pulsed in food processor

1 tablespoon golden monk fruit or brown sugar–style erythritol

1 tablespoon light butter, cut into small pieces

1 Preheat oven to 350°F.

2 Place peaches cut side up on medium baking sheet that's covered in nonstick foil.

3 In a small bowl, combine amaretto, rum, and vanilla and set aside.

4 Sprinkle approximately 1½ teaspoons ground oats into hole and on flesh of each peach, then sprinkle each peach with ½ teaspoon monk fruit.

5 Top each with ½ teaspoon of butter pieces and pour liquor mixture over all peach halves.

6 Bake 20 minutes, then broil 1–2 minutes if a crispier texture is desired. Take care not to burn peaches. Serve.

SERVES 6	
Per Serving:	
Calories	100
Fat	2g
Saturated Fat	1g
Cholesterol	0mg
Sodium	10mg
Carbohydrates	16g
Fiber	2g
Sugar	11g
Added Sugars	2g
Protein	2g

Deconstructed Chocolate-Dipped Apple

SERVES 1

Per Serving:

Calories	200
Fat	7g
Saturated Fat	3.5g
Cholesterol	0mg
Sodium	50mg
Carbohydrates	35g
Fiber	7g
Sugar	25g
Added Sugars	5g
Protein	5g

Chocolate- and candy-coated apples are feel-good boardwalk mainstays. This version has a fraction of the added sugar and calories in a fun, festive treat.

1 medium apple such as Gala, Fuji, or Honeycrisp, cored

½ teaspoon lemon juice

1 teaspoon chopped peanuts

1½ teaspoons unsweetened shredded coconut

1 tablespoon powdered peanut butter

2 teaspoons mini chocolate chips

1 Slice apple into about eighteen slices, place in a small bowl, and toss with lemon juice.

2 Layer apples on a medium plate and sprinkle with peanuts and coconut.

3 In a separate small bowl, add powdered peanut butter and reconstitute with water to desired consistency. Drizzle over apples.

4 Top with chocolate chips and serve.

Peanut Butter Blueberry Snack Squares

These snackable squares resemble a PB and J sandwich with no added sugar. Enjoy one for a quick bite or crumble on top of Greek yogurt for an easy breakfast. They taste even better out of the refrigerator.

1 cup white whole-wheat flour

¾ cup powdered peanut butter

¼ cup plus 1 tablespoon spoonable stevia, divided

1 teaspoon baking powder

1 teaspoon baking soda

1 teaspoon ground cinnamon

1 large egg

2 medium very ripe bananas, mashed

1 teaspoon vanilla extract

2 tablespoons olive oil

½ cup unsweetened applesauce

½ cup plain nonfat Greek yogurt

1¼ cups frozen wild blueberries, divided

1 Preheat oven to 375°F. Line a 9" × 9" square baking pan with parchment paper.

2 In a medium bowl, add flour, powdered peanut butter, ¼ cup plus 2 teaspoons stevia, baking powder, baking soda, and cinnamon and whisk to combine.

3 In a separate medium bowl, beat egg. Add bananas, vanilla, oil, applesauce, and yogurt and combine well.

4 Add wet ingredients to dry ingredients and gently stir until just combined.

5 In a small bowl, combine 1 cup blueberries with remaining 1 teaspoon stevia.

6 Transfer half of batter into prepared pan and distribute evenly.

7 Spread 1 cup blueberries over batter. Add remaining batter and even out the top. Sprinkle on remaining ¼ cup blueberries.

8 Bake 20 minutes or until toothpick inserted in center comes out clean.

9 Let pan cool on a rack, then remove and slice into sixteen squares. Serve and store extras in the refrigerator.

Fig, Ricotta, and Almond Dessert Pizza

SERVES 2

Per Serving:

Calories	160
Fat	6g
Saturated Fat	1.5g
Cholesterol	15mg
Sodium	230mg
Carbohydrates	29g
Fiber	10g
Sugar	17g
Added Sugars	2g
Protein	10g

Sweet summer figs are a precious treat to enjoy on top of this protein- and fiber-packed dessert pizza. If you don't have pure maple syrup, substitute with honey.

1 (8") high-fiber, low-carb flour tortilla
½ cup low-fat ricotta cheese
¼ teaspoon almond extract
2 medium fresh figs, thinly sliced
1 tablespoon sliced almonds
1 teaspoon pure maple syrup

1 Preheat oven to 400°F. Lightly toast tortilla on oven rack 3 minutes.
2 Meanwhile, in a small bowl, mix ricotta cheese and almond extract. Remove tortilla from oven and spread on ricotta mixture.
3 Top with figs and sprinkle with almonds.
4 Toast again approximately 4–5 minutes or until you see steam and cheese is slightly melted. Drizzle with syrup and serve.

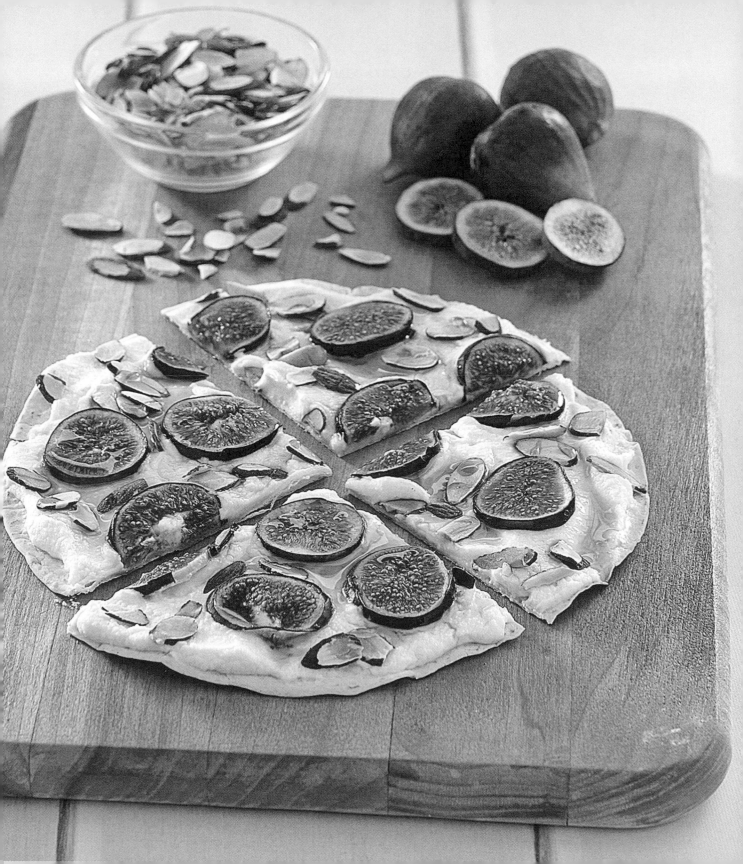

Oven-Roasted Summer Fruit

SERVES 6	
Per Serving:	
Calories	60
Fat	0g
Saturated Fat	0g
Cholesterol	0mg
Sodium	0mg
Carbohydrates	14g
Fiber	3g
Sugar	10g
Added Sugars	0g
Protein	1g

All the sweetness of summer in this easy dessert to please party guests. If you have very ripe, sweet fruit, feel free to leave out the sweetener. It's delicious served with a dollop of light ice cream or vanilla Greek yogurt.

3 medium ripe plums, pitted and quartered

3 medium ripe peaches, pitted and cut into eighths

1 tablespoon spoonable stevia

1 cup raspberries

1 tablespoon orange juice

1 Preheat oven to 450°F.
2 Place peaches and plums in a single layer in a medium ovenproof baking dish. Sprinkle with stevia and top with raspberries.
3 Bake 15–20 minutes until peaches and plums are just tender. Turn on broiler and broil for 3–5 minutes until raspberries release juices.
4 Drizzle with orange juice and serve.

Brownie Batter Hummus Dip

SERVES 6	
Per Serving (¼ cup):	
Calories	150
Fat	6g
Saturated Fat	2.5g
Cholesterol	0mg
Sodium	190mg
Carbohydrates	21g
Fiber	7g
Sugar	6g
Added Sugars	5g
Protein	5g

No one will know that beans are the star of this rich chocolate hummus! Enjoy it as a dip for sliced fruit, as a spread for toast, or by the spoonful to end a meal.

1 (15-ounce) can white beans such as navy or cannellini

¼ cup canned light unsweetened coconut milk

⅓ cup unsweetened cocoa powder

⅓ cup sugar-free maple syrup

1 tablespoon olive oil

1 teaspoon vanilla extract

½ teaspoon kosher salt

¼ cup mini chocolate chips

1 Place all ingredients except chocolate chips into a food processor. Blend until smooth, scraping down the sides as needed.
2 Stir in chocolate chips and serve immediately or cover and refrigerate to thicken. The sweet flavor will increase the longer it sits.

Salt-Free Spice Mixes

Barbecue Blend

- 4 tablespoons dried basil
- 4 tablespoons dried rubbed sage
- 4 tablespoons dried thyme
- 4 teaspoons ground black pepper
- 4 teaspoons dried savory
- 1 teaspoon dried lemon peel

Cajun Blend

- 2 tablespoons ground paprika
- 1 tablespoon garlic powder
- 1 tablespoon onion powder
- ½ tablespoon ground black pepper
- 2 teaspoons ground cayenne pepper
- 2 teaspoons dried oregano
- 2 teaspoons dried thyme

Caribbean Blend

- 1 tablespoon curry powder
- 1 tablespoon ground cumin
- 1 tablespoon ground allspice
- 1 tablespoon ground ginger
- 1 teaspoon ground cayenne pepper

Country Blend

- 5 teaspoons dried thyme
- 4 teaspoons dried basil
- 4 teaspoons dried chervil
- 4 teaspoons dried tarragon

Fish and Seafood Herbs

- 5 teaspoons dried basil
- 5 teaspoons crushed fennel seed
- 4 teaspoons dried parsley
- 1 teaspoon dried lemon peel

French Blend

- 1 tablespoon crushed dried tarragon
- 1 tablespoon crushed dried chervil
- 1 tablespoon onion powder

Herbes de Provence

- 4 teaspoons dried oregano
- 2 teaspoons dried basil
- 2 teaspoons dried sweet marjoram
- 2 teaspoons dried thyme
- 1 teaspoon dried mint
- 1 teaspoon dried rosemary
- 1 teaspoon dried sage
- 1 teaspoon fennel seed
- 1 teaspoon dried lavender (optional)

Italian Blend

- 1 tablespoon crushed dried basil
- 1 tablespoon crushed dried thyme
- 1 tablespoon crushed dried oregano
- 2 tablespoons garlic powder

Middle Eastern Blend

- 1 tablespoon ground coriander
- 1 tablespoon ground cumin
- 1 tablespoon ground turmeric
- 1 teaspoon ground cinnamon
- 1 teaspoon crushed dried mint

Mediterranean Blend

- 1 tablespoon crushed sun-dried tomatoes
- 1 tablespoon dried basil
- 1 teaspoon dried oregano
- 1 teaspoon dried thyme
- 1 tablespoon garlic powder

TIP: If you don't have a food processor, you can freeze the sun-dried tomatoes so they will be easier to crush; however, that adds moisture to the herb blend, so it can't be stored.

Old Bay Seasoning

- 1 tablespoon celery seed
- 1 tablespoon whole black peppercorns
- 6 medium bay leaves
- ½ teaspoon whole cardamom
- ½ teaspoon mustard seed
- 4 whole cloves
- 1 teaspoon sweet Hungarian paprika
- ½ teaspoon ground mace

Pacific Rim

- 1 tablespoon Chinese five-spice powder
- 1 tablespoon ground paprika
- 1 tablespoon ground ginger
- 1 teaspoon ground black pepper

Sonoran Blend

- 1 tablespoon chili powder
- 1 tablespoon ground black pepper
- 1 tablespoon crushed dried oregano
- 1 tablespoon crushed dried thyme
- 1 tablespoon ground coriander
- 1 tablespoon garlic powder

Stuffing Blend

- 6 tablespoons dried rubbed sage
- 3 tablespoons dried sweet marjoram
- 2 tablespoons dried parsley
- 4 teaspoons dried celery flakes

Texas Seasoning

- 3 tablespoons dried cilantro
- 2 tablespoons dried oregano
- 4 teaspoons dried thyme
- 2 tablespoons pure good-quality chili powder
- 2 tablespoons ground black pepper
- 2 tablespoons ground cumin
- 2 small dried chili peppers, crushed
- 1 teaspoon garlic powder

APPENDIX B
Grocery Shopping Pro Tips

Pasta

When choosing pasta, look for those with a high-fiber content. There are several varieties of pasta on the market and each provides slightly different flavors and nutrient info.

- **Whole-grain pasta:** Made with 100 percent whole-wheat or other whole-grain flours with an average of 5 grams of fiber per 2-ounce dry serving, which yields 1 cup cooked.
- **Fiber-enriched pasta:** Isolated fibers are added to the base flour, which increases the total fiber content but with the taste of white flour pasta. The fiber can range from similar to whole wheat to well beyond. Some brands may have up to 20 grams of fiber per 2-ounce dry serving (1 cup cooked). These are usually the most family friendly as they most resemble the appearance and taste of traditional pasta.
- **Bean-based pasta:** These are made from flours derived from beans and legumes such as chickpeas, lentils, edamame, black beans, mung beans, and more. These are gluten free and generally much higher in protein and fiber than wheat pasta though each variety will vary. Expect anywhere from 3–13 grams of fiber per 2-ounce serving with a significant plant-based protein content. They also have unique flavors and don't necessarily taste like traditional pasta.
- **Very low-carb pasta alternatives:** Items such as shirataki made from konjac (a root found in Asia), heart of palm pasta, and "zoodles" (made from zucchini) are becoming more mainstream in supermarkets. These certainly have textures and flavors that differ from what you would expect in pasta, but the calorie and carb counts are negligible—around 0–20 calories per serving with less than 4 grams of carbs. They can taste good when made with interesting sauces, but don't feel the need to eat these unless you really wish to. It's also okay to mix together different pasta varieties for better acceptance. Combine zucchini noodles with whole-grain or bean-based pasta to up the vegetable content and lower total carbs without giving up 100 percent of the pasta you want.

Bread

Sometimes it feels like one needs a PhD in bread science to choose an option to fit your personal taste preferences and dietary needs at the same time. Let's try and make it easier.

For the recipes in this book, look for a bread with 40–50 calories per slice, preferably high in fiber with at least 3 grams or up to 7 grams per slice. You will find these advertised as light wheat, light whole wheat, light whole-grain white, or thin sliced. The whole point here is controlling the carbs. A light bread will generally have half of the carbohydrates of a traditional slice of loaf bread so you can have two slices for the carbs in one. The ingredient lists may be long, and there may be some ingredients you cannot pronounce. Ultimately, you need to choose what works best for you. Some suggested brands are Schmidt Old Tyme 647, Nature's Harvest Light, Nature's Own Life Bread Double Fiber, Alvarado Street Bakery Sprouted Wheat Flaxseed bread, or Silver Hills Bakery Little Big Sprouted Grain Bread. Ezekiel and Dave's Killer Bread are also good options with very simple ingredients but higher calorie counts.

Protein Powder

There are so many different protein powders available that it takes a little experimentation to determine what you like.

Whey

Whey protein powder is a favorite because it has a pleasant flavor and contains the highest amount of protein for the fewest calories. It is also high in the amino acid leucine, which can help with muscle recovery after a workout. Choose a whey protein with very few ingredients sweetened with stevia or monk fruit if you prefer to use the "natural" sweeteners. The varieties used in these recipes provide 20 grams of protein per ¼ cup for 90–120 calories. If you cannot find a similar product or they are out of your price range, don't worry. Other options will still work well, though you may be consuming a few extra calories in carbohydrates in order to achieve the same amount of protein.

Plant-Based (Vegan)

If you prefer a plant-based protein, there are several on the market with similar calorie-to-protein ratios. These are usually some combination of protein from peas, brown rice, cranberry, or soy. They add a bit of a "woodsy" flavor so if you like that, you can certainly switch things up. One thing to note is that plant-based protein powders tend to absorb more liquid so you may have to adjust the recipes when making that substitution, especially if you are letting it sit overnight.

Collagen

New on the scene over the past few years is collagen powder. The calories and carbs are usually similar to that of whey, and the flavor in recipes depends on the type and amount of sweetener used in the powder. It's important to note that there is not a lot of evidence to support any of the advertised benefits of collagen powder and it is not a complete source of protein like whey as it lacks the amino acid tryptophan. If you decide to add collagen to your routine, at best you'll be preserving your youthful skin and promoting joint/bone health, and at worst you'll be taking in some extra protein, according to current research. It is pricey so don't feel you need to use it in lieu of other options.

Plant-Based Milk Alternatives

There is much confusion among consumers with the introduction of milk alternatives like almond, cashew, coconut, and oat milk beverages. People may use them interchangeably with dairy milk, but they are by no means the same. Nut milks have little to no protein, and there are significantly fewer calories and carbohydrates in unsweetened varieties than in cow's milk. The key is choosing the unsweetened ones with no added sugar. Many recipes here use these unsweetened nut milks as a culinary choice, not a moral one. There is no reason to avoid dairy milk unless you have an allergy or intolerance. With pre-diabetes we are monitoring carbohydrate intake, and using these no-added-sugar plant-based milks allows for more of your daily carbohydrate grams to be allocated to fruit or whole grains, which brings more fiber into your diet. Make sure to check that your brand is fortified with calcium and vitamin D, as most organic brands do not fortify nut milks.

Ultra-filtered Milk

Another option is ultra-filtered milk, which is simply milk passed through special filters to concentrate the protein and calcium and remove most of the sugar (lactose). The result is a delicious, creamy milk that has less than 50 percent of the carbohydrate and one and a half times the protein per serving. It's a delicious option for dairy milk lovers and provides that extra protein at breakfast when using it in cereal or coffee. Fairlife is a popular brand.

Oats

Several recipes in this cookbook utilize oats for breakfast entrees or as a flour replacement in baked goods. There are three main types of oats: old-fashioned rolled oats, quick oats, and steel cut oats. They are each subject to a different level of processing with steel cut as the least processed to quick cook oats as the most. To keep it simple, everything in this book uses old-fashioned oats. Quick oats will also work for any recipe that calls for grinding the oats into flour, though steel cut will not. So, if you like steel cut oats, cook them up for a hearty breakfast but refrain from using them in these recipes.

Tortillas and Flatbreads

Many lower-calorie, high-fiber/low-carb options are now available in supermarkets, big box stores, and warehouse clubs. There are many delicious recipes in this book that feature tortillas and flatbreads that contribute significantly fewer calories and carbohydrates than the kind you will find in restaurants and sandwich shops.

Look for flour tortillas that are fajita/taco size with 50–70 calories, and 6–12 grams of fiber for an 8" serving. Some options come in smaller and larger sizes. Your market may display these near the deli, in the bread aisle, in the produce section, with the ethnic foods like taco shells and salsa, or in the dairy aisle. If you are wondering, ask the grocery manager for assistance. Some popular brands are

Mission Carb Balance flour tortillas, Tumaros Carb Wise wraps, La Banderita Carb Counter, La Tortilla Factory Low Carb flour tortillas, Trader Joe's Carb Savvy Tortillas, and Ole Xtreme Wellness tortilla wraps.

Flatbreads that meet carb and fiber guidelines generally have 90–110 calories each with 4–10 grams of fiber. Popular brands are Flatout, Joseph's Flax, Oat Bran and Whole Wheat Lavash and Damascus Bakeries BakeSense Lavash.

A note about gluten-free items: Messages are confusing, but be assured that gluten-free items are not healthier unless you have celiac disease or a documented gluten intolerance. In fact, when it comes to managing blood sugar, they are often less desirable choices. Whole-grain wheat, resistant starch, and wheat starch contain gluten and are often used to add fiber to breads, cereals, and tortillas/flatbreads. Gluten-free versions are typically made from highly refined, low-fiber starches, and may raise blood sugar more.

Your 10-Week Plan to Kick Pre-Diabetes

The 10-Week Plan to Kick Pre-Diabetes is designed to help you set modest goals and put what you have learned into practice. Each week has a healthy lifestyle theme along with some suggested goals to help you achieve success.

Week 1: Check Your Portions

Portion control is key, even when you choose healthy foods! You can have too much of a good thing, and if weight management is onc of your concerns, understanding proper portions is critical to success. One simple approach is to use the plate method. The concept is designed to help you put together healthy meals in appropriate portions and distribute carbohydrates evenly in meals.

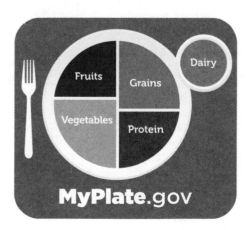

Using the plate method at lunch and dinner, fill ½ of your plate with vegetables, ¼ with starches, and ¼ with lean protein or meat substitute. A serving of dairy/nondairy milk products and fruit are also added to the meal.

Your Goals for Week 1
- Give the plate method a try as a means to reduce portion sizes.
- For several days, measure or weigh your food so you can see just how much you are eating.

Week 2: Eat More Vegetables and Fruits Every Day

The recommendation to eat five to nine servings of fruit and vegetables every day sounds like a lot of food, but once you know how to incorporate these foods into your plan it becomes easy. Why that many servings? Because fruit and vegetables are nutrient-dense foods that are high in fiber and low in calories. Plus, the antioxidants and phytochemicals in produce can play a role in improving insulin resistance.

Your Goals for Week 2

- Take two pieces of fruit from home each day to have for a snack or with lunch.
- Keep raw vegetables washed, cut up, and ready to eat for quick snacks or salads. If they are there, you will eat them!

Week 3: Get Walking!

No matter how long you are able to walk, doing it consistently is most important. Aim for walking most days of the week. Make sure that you have comfortable walking shoes or sneakers.

Your Goals for Week 3

- Walk for as long as you are comfortable. Keep a written record of when and how long you are walking.
- Wear a pedometer or fitness tracker, or use an app on your phone to monitor how many steps you take each day. Use the number as a motivator to help you increase your steps each day.

Week 4: Switch to Whole Grains

Begin to switch out the white flour and refined white grain products in your kitchen for whole-grain foods. Whole grains provide more fiber and nutrients and have less impact on your blood glucose. Look for products that list whole-grain flour rather than enriched flour as one of the first ingredients. Also look for higher-fiber versions of items you already use.

Your Goals for Week 4

- Add whole-grain pasta or brown rice to a favorite dish or in combination with vegetables or beans.
- Purchase a new whole-grain food that you haven't used before and try it as a replacement for rice, pasta, or potatoes. Some suggestions: quinoa, kasha, wild rice, sorghum, farro, or bulgur.

Week 5: Manage Your Stress

Take stress seriously and find ways to reduce it. Chronic stress can wreak havoc on health and well-being by lowering your immunity and making you more susceptible to many types of illness. Plus, stress hormones can contribute to weight gain. You are working on ways to halt prediabetes in its tracks; don't let stress derail you!

Your Goals for Week 5

- Add stretching exercises, meditation, or deep breathing exercises to your daily routine.
- Allow yourself some downtime from the daily grind each day that doesn't include screens. Make this time for yourself by choosing a relaxing activity that you enjoy.

Week 6: Get Adequate Sleep

Insufficient sleep can have a negative impact on your health. Research has shown that poor-quality sleep on a regular basis can contribute to insulin resistance, metabolic syndrome, and diabetes—just what you are trying to avoid!

Your Goals for Week 6

- Even if you are very busy or have a demanding schedule, resist the urge to skimp on sleep. Make enough time to get seven to eight hours of sleep each night.
- Develop good sleeping habits by rising and retiring at about the same time each day. Avoid TV and cell phone screens an hour before bed to allow your brain to prepare for sleep. If you have trouble settling your mind, try going to sleep listening to an app that plays soothing sounds.

Week 7: Don't Forget the Snacks

Having meals and snacks at regular times can go a long way toward controlling your appetite and blood glucose. Snacking during the day is fine, as long as you make good choices that are rich in nutrients and low in calories. Always try to pair a source of protein and healthy fat with your carbohydrate foods.

Goals for Week 7

- When grocery shopping, buy healthy snacks to have on hand at all times.
- Come up with at least two new snack options this week to prevent boredom.
- If necessary, prepare snacks ahead of time, so they are always ready to go (e.g., cut up vegetables, pre-measure nuts into individual containers/baggies, and so on).

Week 8: Ramp Up Your Exercise

You may have started an exercise plan several weeks ago, but it's time to take it up a notch. This is important because exercising the same muscles or at the same intensity all of the time will eventually stall your efforts at weight loss. Strength training is important to assist with building and maintaining muscle mass that uses up more glucose and calories.

Goals for Week 8

- Turn your moderate walk into a brisk walk. Step up the pace of your walk and add additional steps by using your step tracker to measure your progress.
- Add a few flexibility or strength training exercises to your routine in addition to walking.

Week 9: Change Your Food Behaviors

Negative food habits are not always easy to change. Make a conscious effort to improve eating habits that may be inhibiting your progress toward your health goals.

Goals for Week 9

- Pay attention to your hunger. Try to eat when you actually feel hungry and stop when you no longer feel hungry versus when you have cleared your plate.

- Slow down when you eat. Fast eating or mindless/distracted eating can cause you to eat too much food before you realize that you've had enough. Place your fork down between each bite and allow more time to eat your meal or snack.
- Drink plenty of water. Take a water bottle with you wherever you go, set one on your desk at work, or find ways to remind yourself to drink more water. Most people need about 64–96 ounces of fluid a day; make most of it water!

Week 10: Progress Check

Monitor your overall progress by looking at how well you have done with various aspects of your plan.

Goals for Week 10

- Make a list of all of the things you have been able to achieve, as well as the goals that you are working on.
- Seeing in writing all that you have accomplished is very satisfying and motivates you to keep going. Congratulate and reward yourself for a job well done!

STANDARD US/METRIC MEASUREMENT CONVERSIONS

WEIGHT CONVERSIONS

US Weight Measure	Metric Equivalent
½ ounce	15 grams
1 ounce	30 grams
2 ounces	60 grams
3 ounces	85 grams
¼ pound (4 ounces)	115 grams
½ pound (8 ounces)	225 grams
¾ pound (12 ounces)	340 grams
1 pound (16 ounces)	454 grams

VOLUME CONVERSIONS

US Volume Measure	Metric Equivalent
⅛ teaspoon	0.5 milliliter
¼ teaspoon	1 milliliter
½ teaspoon	2 milliliters
1 teaspoon	5 milliliters
½ tablespoon	7 milliliters
1 tablespoon (3 teaspoons)	15 milliliters
2 tablespoons (1 fluid ounce)	30 milliliters
¼ cup (4 tablespoons)	60 milliliters
⅓ cup	90 milliliters
½ cup (4 fluid ounces)	125 milliliters
⅔ cup	160 milliliters
¾ cup (6 fluid ounces)	180 milliliters
1 cup (16 tablespoons)	250 milliliters
1 pint (2 cups)	500 milliliters
1 quart (4 cups)	1 liter (about)

OVEN TEMPERATURE CONVERSIONS

Degrees Fahrenheit	Degrees Celsius
200 degrees F	95 degrees C
250 degrees F	120 degrees C
275 degrees F	135 degrees C
300 degrees F	150 degrees C
325 degrees F	160 degrees C
350 degrees F	180 degrees C
375 degrees F	190 degrees C
400 degrees F	205 degrees C
425 degrees F	220 degrees C
450 degrees F	230 degrees C

BAKING PAN SIZES

American	Metric
8 × 1½ inch round baking pan	20 × 4 cm cake tin
9 × 1½ inch round baking pan	23 × 3.5 cm cake tin
11 × 7 × 1½ inch baking pan	28 × 18 × 4 cm baking tin
13 × 9 × 2 inch baking pan	30 × 20 × 5 cm baking tin
2 quart rectangular baking dish	30 × 20 × 3 cm baking tin
15 × 10 × 2 inch baking pan	30 × 25 × 2 cm baking tin (Swiss roll tin)
9 inch pie plate	22 × 4 or 23 × 4 cm pie plate
7 or 8 inch springform pan	18 or 20 cm springform or loose bottom cake tin
9 × 5 × 3 inch loaf pan	23 × 13 × 7 cm or 2 lb narrow loaf or pate tin
1½ quart casserole	1.5 liter casserole
2 quart casserole	2 liter casserole

Index

Improve your health and lower your risk of type 2 diabetes!

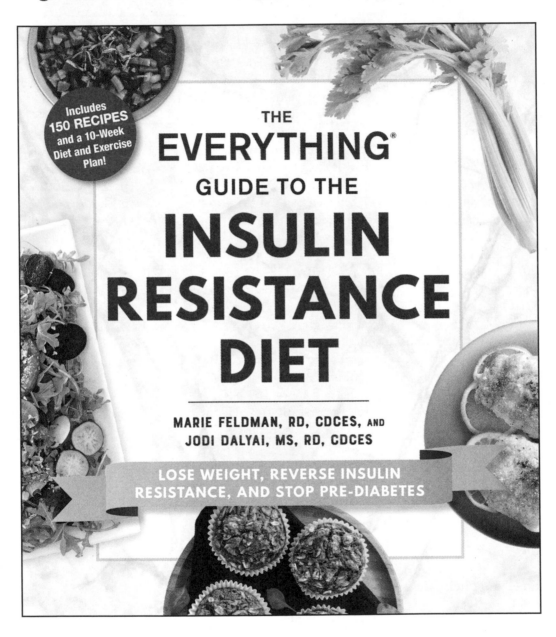

Includes 150 RECIPES and a 10-Week Diet and Exercise Plan!

THE

EVERYTHING®
GUIDE TO THE
INSULIN RESISTANCE DIET

MARIE FELDMAN, RD, CDCES, AND
JODI DALYAI, MS, RD, CDCES

LOSE WEIGHT, REVERSE INSULIN
RESISTANCE, AND STOP PRE-DIABETES

PICK UP OR DOWNLOAD YOUR COPY TODAY!

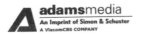
adamsmedia
An Imprint of Simon & Schuster
A ViacomCBS COMPANY